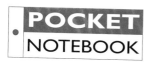

POCKET
NOTEBOOK

Pocket
FOOT AND
ANKLE
MEDICINE
AND SURGERY

T0200318

Edited by

ROCK G. POSITANO, DPM, MSc, MPH
Director and Founder of the Non-Surgical Foot and Ankle Service
Hospital for Special Surgery
Joe DiMaggio Sports Medicine Foot and Ankle Center
Sports Medicine Service
Weill Cornell Medicine
Department of Medicine–Division of Endocrinology, Diabetes and Metabolism
Department of Cardiothoracic Surgery
Department of Obstetrics and Gynecology
Memorial Sloan Kettering Cancer Center (MSKCC)
Orthopedic Service/Foot and Ankle Division/Department of Surgery
Lenox Hill Hospital
Professor
New York College of Podiatric Medicine/Foot Center of New York
Departments of Academic Orthopedic Science/Medicine/Orthopedics
New York, New York

CHRISTOPHER W. DiGIOVANNI, MD
Associate Professor & Vice Chairman (Academic Affairs)
Harvard Medical School
Chief, Division of Foot & Ankle Surgery
Director, Harvard-MGH Foot and Ankle Fellowship Program
Department of Orthopaedic Surgery
Massachusetts General Hospital and Newton-Wellesley Hospital
Boston, Massachusetts
MGH-NWH Foot & Ankle Center
Waltham, Massachusetts

ANDREW J. ROSENBAUM, MD
Assistant Professor
Director of Orthopaedic Research
Division of Orthopaedic Surgery
Albany Medical College
Albany, New York

RONALD L. SOAVE, DPM, FACFAS
Chair, Department of Medicine and Professor of Surgery
New York College of Podiatric Medicine
New York, New York
Past Chief and Residency Director
New York-Presbyterian Brooklyn Methodist Hospital
Brooklyn, New York
Diplomate
American Board of Foot and Ankle Surgery
San Francisco, California
Diplomate
American Board of Podiatric Medicine
Hermosa Beach, California
Fellow
American College of Foot and Ankle Surgeons
Chicago, Illinois

NORMAN A. WORTZMAN, DPM, FACFAOM
Lead Podiatrist
Division of Foot and Ankle Surgery
Department of Orthopaedic Surgery
Massachusetts General Hospital
Boston, Massachusetts
Diplomate
American Board of Podiatric Medicine
Hermosa Beach, California
Fellow
American College of Foot and Ankle Orthopedics and Medicine
Bethesda, Maryland
Associate Member
American Academy of Podiatric Sports Medicine
Ocala, Florida

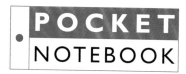

POCKET
NOTEBOOK

Pocket FOOT AND ANKLE MEDICINE AND SURGERY

Edited by

ROCK G. POSITANO, DPM, MSc, MPH

CHRISTOPHER W. DiGIOVANNI, MD

ANDREW J. ROSENBAUM, MD

RONALD L. SOAVE, DPM, FACFAS

NORMAN A. WORTZMAN, DPM, FACFAOM

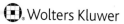. Wolters Kluwer

Philadelphia • Baltimore • New York • London
Buenos Aires • Hong Kong • Sydney • Tokyo

Acquisitions Editor: Brian Brown
Editorial Coordinator: David Murphy
Editorial Assistant: Amy Masgay
Marketing Manager: Julie Sikora
Production Project Manager: Kim Cox
Design Coordinator: Elaine Kasmer
Manufacturing Coordinator: Beth Welsh
Prepress Vendor: S4Carlisle Publishing Services

Copyright © 2019 Wolters Kluwer.

9 8 7 6 5 4 3 2 1

Printed in China

Library of Congress Cataloging-in-Publication Data

Names: Positano, Rock G., editor. | DiGiovanni, Christopher W., editor. | Rosenbaum, Andrew J., editor. | Soave, Ronald L., editor. | Wortzman, Norman A., editor.

Title: Pocket foot and ankle medicine and surgery / [edited by] Rock G. Positano, Christopher W. DiGiovanni, Andrew J. Rosenbaum, Ronald L. Soave, Norman A. Wortzman.

Description: Philadelphia: Wolters Kluwer Health, [2019]

Identifiers: LCCN 2017056380 | ISBN 9781496375292

Subjects: | MESH: Foot Diseases—diagnosis | Foot Diseases—therapy | Foot Injuries—diagnosis | Foot Injuries—therapy | Ankle Injuries—diagnosis | Ankle Injuries—therapy | Orthopedic Procedures—methods | Handbooks

Classification: LCC RD781 | NLM WE 39 | DDC 617.5/85059—dc23

LC record available at https://lccn.loc.gov/2017056380

LWW.com

DEDICATION

I would like to dedicate this to all the medical students, residents, fellows, and other trainees and providers who help us administer musculoskeletal care. I hope they find this book useful.

—CHRISTOPHER DIGIOVANNI

This book is dedicated to my wife Heidi and my three sons, Brett, Jared, and Ethan, who inspire me toward excellence on a daily basis. It is also dedicated to my teachers at the New York College of Podiatric Medicine for setting me along the path to where I am today. Last, it is dedicated to my authors who put up with my deadlines and critiques of their chapters along the way.

—NORMAN WORTZMAN

I would like to dedicate this book to my amazing wife Kristin and my daughters Charlotte and Madison. It is only with your patience, support, and love that I can participate in projects like this. This text is also for my mentors, Scott Ellis and Martin O'Malley, who have had a tremendous impact on my training and career, and who I can only hope to emulate each day. And last, to the students, resident, fellows, and other trainees who regularly challenge me to improve and learn—this book is for you.

—ANDREW ROSENBAUM

I am grateful for the research support of the Stavros Niarchos Foundation, Rudin Family Foundation, James Family Charitable Foundation, and the Heckscher Foundation.

I am so appreciative of the dedication and contributions of my colleagues at the Hospital for Special Surgery, New York-Presbyterian Hospital, Yale School of Public Health, Weill Cornell Medical, Memorial Sloan Kettering Cancer Center, and the New York College of Podiatric Medicine.

The importance of mobility and how it affects the patient's quality of life can never be underestimated. We educate health providers to best serve the needs of the patients, and we dedicate our efforts to this group.

—ROCK POSITANO

I dedicate this book to my parents, wife, and children for their understanding. I am forever grateful to Drs. Jacob and Oloff for the wisdom they bestowed on me and to Dr. Pacella for his mentorship.

—RONALD SOAVE

CONTRIBUTING AUTHORS

Mostafa M. Abousayed, MD, MSc
Resident
Department of Orthopedic Surgery
Albany Medical College
Albany, New York

Konstantin Agarunov, DPM
Chief Resident
Department of Podiatric Medicine and Surgery
Wyckoff Heights Medical Center
Brooklyn, New York

Maxwell C. Alley, BA
MD Candidate Class of 2018
Albany Medical College
Albany, New York

Hanya Almudallal, DPM, AACFAS
Resident
Department of Podiatric Medicine & Surgery
New York-Presbyterian Brooklyn Methodist Hospital
Brooklyn, New York

David G. Armstrong, DPM, MD, PhD
Professor of Surgery and Director
Southwestern Academic Limb Salvage Alliance (SALSA)
Keck School of Medicine of University of Southern California (USC)
Los Angeles, California

Scott T. Bleazey, DPM
Foot and Ankle Surgeon
MidJersey Orthopaedics
Flemington, New Jersey

Cory P. Clement, DPM, AACFAS, DABPM
ACFAS Fellow Physician (2017-18)
Encino Specialty Surgery Center Sports Medicine Fellowship
Los Angeles, California

Matthew R. DiCaprio, MD
Associate Professor
Division of Orthopaedic Surgery
Director of Orthopaedic Oncology
Albany Medical Center
Albany, New York

Christopher W. DiGiovanni, MD
Associate Professor & Vice Chairman (Academic Affairs)
Harvard Medical School
Chief, Division of Foot & Ankle Surgery
Director, Harvard-MGH Foot and Ankle Fellowship Program
Department of Orthopaedic Surgery
Massachusetts General Hospital and Newton-Wellesley Hospital
Boston, Massachusetts
MGH-NWH Foot & Ankle Center
Waltham, Massachusetts

John A. DiPreta, MD
Clinical Associate Professor
Capital Region Orthopaedics
Albany Medical College
Albany, New York

Tonya L. Dixon, MD, MPH
Assistant Professor
Foot and Ankle Surgery
Department of Orthopaedic Surgery
University of Cincinnati
Academic Health Center
Cincinnati, Ohio

Aleksandr Emerel, DPM
House Staff
Department of Foot and Ankle Surgery
Broadlawns Medical Center
Des Moines, Iowa

Yoshimi Endo, MD
Assistant Attending Radiologist
Hospital for Special Surgery
Assistant Professor of Radiology
Weill Cornell Medical College
New York, New York

Satwinder Kaur Gosal, DPM
Podiatrist
Complete Spine and
    Pain Care
Framingham, Massachusetts

Ronald M. Guberman, DPM
Director, Podiatry Residency
    Program
Wyckoff Heights
    Medical Center
Brooklyn, New York

Daniel Guss, MD, MBA
Assistant Professor, Harvard
    Medical School
Foot and Ankle Service
Department of Orthopaedic
    Surgery
Massachusetts General Hospital
Boston, Massachusetts
Newton-Wellesley Hospital
Newton, Massachusetts

David C. Hatch Jr, DPM
Resident
Tucson Medical Center
Tucson, Arizona

Dina Ibrahim, DPM
Foot and Ankle Surgeon
Department of Surgery
New York-Presbyterian Brooklyn
    Methodist Hospital
Brooklyn, New York

Carl M. Jean, DPM, FACFAS
Teaching Faculty
Department of Surgery,
    Podiatry Division
New York-Presbyterian Brooklyn
    Methodist Hospital
Brooklyn, New York

Anne Holly Johnson, MD
Department of Orthopedic
    Surgery
Foot and Ankle Specialist
Massachusetts General Hospital
Harvard Medical School
Boston, Massachusetts

Christopher K. Johnson, MS
Student
Albany Medical College
Albany, New York

**Patrick Jordan, DPM,
    AACFAS**
Attending
SynergyHealth Foot and Ankle
Midlothian, Virginia

Jillian M. Kazley, MD
Resident
Department of Orthopaedic
    Surgery
Albany Medical Center
Albany, New York

Stuart E. Kigner, DPM
Podiatrist
Division of Foot and Ankle
    Surgery
Department of Orthopaedic
    Surgery
Massachusetts General
    Hospital
Boston, Massachusetts
Diplomate
American Board of Podiatric
    Medicine
Hermosa Beach, California

Shaun A. Kink, MD
Orthopedic Surgeon
McLean County Orthopedics
Bloomington, Illinois

Edward Lee, DPM
Attending Surgeon
St. Joseph Medical Center
Houston, Texas
Private Practice
Neville Foot and Ankle
    Centers
The Woodlands, Texas

Jordan M. Lisella, MD
Capital Region Orthopaedics
Assistant Professor
Department of Orthopaedics
Albany Medical Center
Albany, New York

Anthony P. Mechrefe, MD, FAAOS
Clinical Assistant Professor
Department of Family Medicine
Brown University/Warren Alpert
Medical School
Partner
Orthopedics Rhode Island
Warwick, Rhode Island

Nasef Mohamed Nasef, MD
Professor of Orthopedic Surgery
Reconstructive Foot and Ankle
Surgery Consultant
Beni Suef University Teaching
Hospitals
Beni Suef, Cairo, Egypt

Robert L. Parisien, MD
Resident
Department of Orthopaedic Surgery
Boston University School of
Medicine and Medical Center
Boston, Massachusetts

Samuel Parmar, DPM
Associate Director
Department of Podiatry Surgery
New York-Presbyterian Brooklyn
Methodist Hospital
Brooklyn, New York

Rock C. J. Positano, DPM
Resident
Division of Podiatry
The Foot and Ankle Center
New York-Presbyterian Brooklyn
Methodist Hospital
Brooklyn, New York

Rock G. Positano, DPM, MSc, MPH
Director and Founder of the Non-
Surgical Foot and Ankle Service
Hospital for Special Surgery
Joe DiMaggio Sports Medicine
Foot and Ankle Center
Sports Medicine Service
Weill Cornell Medicine
Department of Medicine–Division
of Endocrinology, Diabetes and
Metabolism
Department of Cardiothoracic
Surgery
Department of Obstetrics and
Gynecology
Memorial Sloan Kettering Cancer
Center (MSKCC)
Orthopedic Service/Foot and
Ankle Division/Department
of Surgery
Lenox Hill Hospital
Professor
New York College of Podiatric
Medicine/Foot Center of
New York
Departments of Academic
Orthopedic Science/
Medicine/Orthopedics
New York, New York

Andrew J. Rosenbaum, MD
Assistant Professor
Director of Orthopaedic Research
Division of Orthopaedic Surgery
Albany Medical College
Albany, New York

Manoj Sadhnani, DPM
Associate Professor
Department of Podiatry
New York-Presbyterian Brooklyn
Methodist Hospital
Brooklyn, New York

Ross M. Senter, DPM
Chief Resident
Department of Surgery – Podiatry
New York-Presbyterian Brooklyn
Methodist Hospital
Brooklyn, New York

Ronald L. Soave, DPM, FACFAS
Chair, Department of Medicine
and Professor of Surgery
New York College of Podiatric
Medicine
New York, New York

Past Chief and Residency Director
New York-Presbyterian Brooklyn
    Methodist Hospital
Brooklyn, New York
Diplomate
American Board of Foot and
    Ankle Surgery
San Francisco, California
Diplomate
American Board of Podiatric
    Medicine
Hermosa Beach, California
Fellow
American College of Foot and
    Ankle Surgeons
Chicago, Illinois

Jason P. Tartaglione, MD
Fellow, Foot and Ankle Surgery
Department of Orthopaedic
    Surgery
MedStar Union Memorial Hospital
Baltimore, Maryland

Winston L. Trope
Undergraduate, AB and BE Pending
Thayer School of Engineering
Dartmouth College
Hanover, New Hampshire

Jared Wortzman, MD
Resident
Department of Anesthesia,
    Critical Care and Pain Medicine
Massachusetts General Hospital
Boston, Massachusetts

Norman A. Wortzman, DPM,
    FACFAOM
Lead Podiatrist
Division of Foot and Ankle
    Surgery
Department of Orthopaedic
    Surgery
Massachusetts General
    Hospital
Boston, Massachusetts
Diplomate
American Board of Podiatric
    Medicine
Hermosa Beach, California
Fellow
American College of Foot and
    Ankle Orthopedics and
    Medicine
Bethesda, Maryland
Associate Member
American Academy of Podiatric
    Sports Medicine
Ocala, Florida

Scott Yates, DPM
Podiatrist
Division of Foot and Ankle
    Surgery
Department of Orthopaedic
    Surgery
Massachusetts General Hospital
Boston, Massachusetts
Diplomate
American Board of Podiatric
    Medicine
Hermosa Beach, California

PREFACE

This edition of *Pocket Foot and Ankle Medicine and Surgery* is designed for trainees, clinicians, and allied health specialists focused on the care of patients with conditions affecting the foot and ankle. This text reflects the most current approaches to the diagnosis and treatment of these often complex and challenging disorders. It is designed to be a "pocket" reference that will facilitate effective, evidence-based care. We believe you will find this resource beneficial as you care for your patients.

ANDREW ROSENBAUM

ROCK POSITANO

CHRISTOPHER DIGIOVANNI

NORMAN WORTZMAN

RONALD SOAVE

CONTENTS

STUART E. KIGNER

JOINTS

- **Ankle:** Talus trochlear, medial malleolus, lateral malleolus, tibial plafond
- **Distal tibiofibular joint**—tibia: Incisura fibularis (triangular base distal usually concave), fibula (convex)
  Stabilized by: Syndesmosis—anterior inferior tibiofibular ligament, posterior inferior tibiofibular ligament, interosseous ligament, transverse ligament (deep PITFL), interosseous membrane; **medial**—deltoid superficial, deep ligament; **lateral**—anterior talofibular ligament, calcaneofibular ligament, posterior talofibular ligament
- **Subtalar joint:** Torque dissipator—eversion-inversion of calcaneus converts to int/ext rotation of the leg; pronation-shock absorption, unlocks midtarsal joint—adapts to uneven terrain; supination—locks midtarsal joint allowing foot to function as rigid lever
  Sinus tarsus—space between calcaneus anterior process and talus lateral process
- **Talonavicular joint:** May be considered a gliding ellipsoid joint as the talar head may partially displace out of the navicular acetabulum
- **Midtarsal joint (Chopart joint)**; talonavicular, calcaneocuboid joints
- **Tarsal metatarsal (Lisfranc) joints**—dsfx/plfx degrees range of motion: 1st 3.5, 2nd 0.6, 3rd 1.6, 4th 9.6, 5th 10.2 (*FAI* 1989;10:143), 2nd metatarsal base recessed relative to 1st and 3rd—articulates with five bones, trapezoid shape of met bases 2, 3, 4 forms arch increasing stability of the midfoot (*AAOS Instr Course Lectures*, 2009, p. 185)
- **MTP joints:** 1st—gliding hinge joint (hallux proximal phalanx glides over 1st met head), 2nd to 5th—static stabilization by collateral ligaments, plantar plate, and deep transverse metatarsal ligament. No muscles attach to metatarsal heads.
- **Digits interphalangeal joints:** Hinge-dsflx, plfx, static stabilization collateral ligament
- **Essential joints:** Ankle (tibiotalar), subtalar, talonavicular, cuboid metatarsal, MTP (*Core Knowledge in Orthopaedics-DiGiovanni CW*, 2007, p. 4)

BONES

- **Tibia:** Plafond-concave medial/lateral and anterior/post, distal lateral-incisura fibularis, medial malleolus-anterior, post colliculi, malleolar groove (tib post tendon)
- **Fibula:** Lateral malleolus—approx 1 cm post and lateral to medial malleolus, retromalleolar groove (peroneus brevis-deep, peroneus longus-superficial)
- **Talus**—no muscular/tendon attachment; 2/3 cartilage; **head** (articulates navicular); **neck; body:** Dome (trochlear) wider anteriorly, posterior facet, groove for FHL between post medial and post lateral tubercles (Stieda-elongated post lateral process); lateral process-attach ATFL, PTFL, lateral talocalc; medial surface-articular, deltoid attach
- **Calcaneus:** Superior-anterior facet, middle facet (above sustentaculum tali), post facet (largest); plantar-medial, lateral tubercles; post-tuberosity; medial-sustentaculum tali (support talar neck, inferior aspect-groove FHL); lateral-peroneal tubercle (peroneus brevis-superior, peroneus longus inferior); anterior-articular surface, anterior process (origin-bifurcate ligament); neutral triangle-trabeculae void, under talar lateral process
- **Cuboid:** Plantar-groove (peroneus longus)
- **Navicular:** Tuberosity-primary insertion of tibialis posterior, attachment of spring ligament
- **Cuneiforms:** Wedge shape, medial cuneiform-base plantar, intermediate and lateral-base dorsal
- **Metatarsal**—head, shaft, base; **1st:** metatarsal head plantar-crista (ridge separating grooves overlying sesamoids); **5th**-tuberosity-insertion of peroneus brevis, apophysis proximal
- **Metatarsal (length):** 2>3>1>4>5 (*Sarrafian's Anatomy of Foot and Ankle*, 3rd ed, p. 81), 1st intermetatarsal angle 3° to 9°, metatarsal inclination angle decreases met1→5
- **Sesamoids:** Medial: conjoint tendons-abductor hallucis, FHB, lateral: conjoint tendon-add hallucis, FHB; FHL tendons located between sesamoids; often bipartite; dorsal articulation with 1st metatarsal head
- **Phalanges:** 5th toe distal and middle phalanx coalition (synostosis) common
- **Forefoot**—phalanges, metatarsals; **Midfoot**-navicular, cuneiform, cuboid; **Rearfoot**-calcaneus, talus
- **Longitudinal arch: Medial**-calcaneus, talus, navicular, cuneiforms, metatarsal 1,2,3; **Lateral**-calcaneus, cuboid, metatarsal 4,5. **Transverse arch:** Cuboid, cuneiforms, adjacent metatarsals 1 to 5 (*McMinn's Foot & Ankle Anatomy*, 4th ed, p. 51)

- **Columns: Medial**-talus, navicular, medial cuneiform, 1st metatarsal; **lateral**-calcaneus, cuboid metatarsals 4,5
- **Ray:** 1,2,3-metatarsal+cuneiform, 4,5 metatarsal alone

MUSCLES/TENDONS

- **Achilles tendon:** Hypovascular 2 to 6 cm proximal to insertion; gastroc fibers rotate from post to post/lateral or laterally from proximal to distal; surrounded by peritenon (no synovial sheath); insertion-posterior calcaneus
- **Tibialis anterior:** Passes deep to upper and lower segments of inferior extensor retinaculum; insertion medial surface medial cuneiform, inferomedial 1st met base
- **Tibialis posterior:** Under flexor retinaculum 1st compartment; insertion-navicular tuberosity, cuneiform 1,2,3, cuboid, met base 2,3,4, calcaneus, hypovascular 2.2 to 1.5 cm proximal to medial mal (FAI 36:436-443)
- **FDL:** Flexor retinaculum 2nd compartment, under plantar plate deep to FDB, insertion base of distal phalanx 2 to 5
- **FHL:** Flexor retinaculum 4th compartment; under plantar plate between sesamoids; insertion base of distal phalanx hallux
- **FDB:** Origin-medial calcaneal tubercle, plantar fascia; divides at base proximal phalanx; inserts middle phalanx 2 to 5
- **FHB:** Insert-base proximal phalanx, sesamoids, plantar plate
- **EDL:** Under superior extensor retinaculum divides into two tendons, just distal to inferior extensor retinaculum each tendon divides into two tendons; EDB tendons join laterally at MTP joint, lumbricals join medially, insert middle and distal phalanges
- **EDB:** Insert lateral EDL 1 to 4, only muscle dorsum of foot
- **Peroneus tertius:** Under extensor retinaculum insert dorsal base 5th met
- **Peroneus longus:** Posterior to peroneus brevis in peroneal groove, inferior to peroneus brevis over lateral calcaneus; inferior lateral cuboid—os peroneum; insertion 1st met base plantar lateral, plantar medial cuneiform
- **Peroneus brevis:** Insertion tuberosity of 5th metatarsal
- **Interossei:** Dorsal to deep transverse intermetatarsal ligament; plantar to MTP joint axis; three plantar adduct phalanges 3,4,5; four dorsal abduct phalanges 2,3,4
- **Lumbricals:** Origin FDL; plantar to transverse intermetatarsal ligament; plantar to MTP joint axis
- **Extensor hood: Sling** (proximal) fibroaponeurotic structure anchoring extensor tendons at MTP and proximal

phalanx, extends around MTP joint capsule joining plantar plate, flexor tendon sheath, deep transverse metatarsal ligament (*Sarrafian's Anatomy of the Foot and Ankle*, 3rd ed, p. 229), **wing** (distal), covers base of lesser toes and MTP joints; Extensor apparatus: EDL, EDB, lumbrical, interossei, extensor sling, extensor wing, triangular laminar

- **Master knot of Henry:** FDL (superficial) crosses over FHL (deep), fibrous sling, plantar to navicular, allows independent excursion

LAYERS ON THE SOLE OF THE FOOT

- **1st:** Abductor hallucis, flexor digitorum brevis, abductor digiti minimi
- **2nd:** Quadratus plantae, lumbricals, tendons of FDL, FHL
- **3rd:** Flexor halluces brevis, adductor halluces, flexor digiti minimi brevis
- **4th:** Interossei, tendons of tibialis posterior, fibularis (peroneus) longus

Muscles of the Foot and Ankle

Muscle	Origin	Insertion	Function
Gastrocnemius	Femur-medial and lateral condyles	Achilles tendon	Ankle plfx STJ-sup
Soleus	Tibia-upper fibular-posterior upper	Achilles tendon	Ankle plfx STJ-sup
Plantaris	Femur-lateral supracondylar line	Posterior calcaneus, medial achilles	Ankle plfx STJ-sup
Tibialis posterior	Tibia, fibular medial	Navicular tuberosity, cuneiform 1,2,3 met base 2,3,4 cuboid calcaneus	Ankle-plfx STJ-sup
Flexor digitorum longus	Tibia medial posterior	Digits 2–5, plantar distal phalanx base	Ankle-plfx STJ-sup MTP-plfx
Flexor hallucis longus	Fibular-2/3 post surface	Hallux plantar distal phalanx base	Ankle-plfx STJ-sup MTP-plfx

Muscles of the Foot and Ankle (*continued*)

Muscle	Origin	Insertion	Function
Tibialis anterior	Tibia-lateral upper 2/3	1st met base-medial cuneiform, inferomedial	Ankle-dsfx STJ-sup
Extensor hallucis longus	Fibular-medial middle 1/3	Hallux dorsal distal phalanx base	Ankle-dsfx STJ-neutral MTP-dsfx
Extensor digitorum longus	Anterior fibular, tibia	Digit 2-5: dorsal distal and middle phalanx	Ankle-dsfx STJ-pronator MTP-dsfx
Fibularis (peroneus) tertius	Fibular anterior surface	5th met base-dorsal	Ankle-dsfx STJ-pronation
Fibularis (peroneus) longus	Fibular-lateral surface upper 2/3	1st met base lateral medial cuneiform	Ankle-plfx STJ-pronation 1st ray plfx
Fibularis (peroneus) brevis	Fibular lateral surface-lower 2/3	5th met base-lateral	Ankle-dsfx STJ-pronation
Extensor digitorum brevis	Calcaneus	Hallux base prox phalanx, dorsal digital expansion digits 2-4	MTP-1-4 dsfx
Abductor hallucis	Calcaneus-medial tuberosity	Hallux proximal phalanx medial base	1st MTP plfx, abd
Flexor digitorum brevis	Calcaneus-medial tuberosity	Digits 2–4: middle phalanx	MTP-2-4 plfx PIP 2-4 plfx
Abductor digiti minimi	Calcaneus-medial lateral tuberosity	5th toe proximal phalanx lateral base	5th mtp plfx, adb
Quadratus plantae (flexor accessorius)	Calcaneus-medial surface, plantar calcaneus	Flexor digitorum longus tendons	MTP 2-4 plfx

(*continued*)

Muscles of the Foot and Ankle (continued)

Muscle	Origin	Insertion	Function
Lumbricals	Flexor digitorum longus tendons	EDL tendon digital expansion	MTP 2-4 plfx IP extension
Flexor hallucis brevis	Cuboid, lateral cuneiform plantar surface	Great toe prox phalanx base medial and lateral	1st MTj-plfx
Adductor hallucis	Oblique head: 2nd–4th met base transverse head: toes 3-5 MTPj ligament	Great toe-lateral base prox phalanx	Great toe-adduction
Flexor digiti minimi brevis	5th met base-plantar	5th toe-prox phalanx base-lateral	5th MTPj-plfx
Interosseus dorsal	Adjacent sides of metatarsal shafts	First-medial prox phalanx 2nd toe, 2,3,4-lateral prox phalanx toes 2,3,4	Toes 2–4, MTPj plfx, extension Ipj
Interosseus plantar	Base, medial side metatarsal 3–5	Prox phalanx medial base 3–5	Toes 3-5 MTPj plfx, extension Ipj

LIGAMENTS

- **Ankle-lateral:** Anterior talofibular (anterior surface lateral mal-talar body), calcaneofibular (anterior surface lateral mal-lateral calc, extracapsular), post talofibular (medial surface lateral mal-post talus)
- **Ankle-medial: Deltoid: deep** -deep posterior tibiotalar-thickest band (origin: tibia intercollicular groove-insertion: medial talar body),deep ant tibiotalar(origin: inferior anterior medial malleolus-insertion: medial talar body; **superficial**-tibionavicular (origin: medial malleolus ant colliculus-insertion: dorsal medial navicular), tibiospring (origin: ant tibial colliculus-insertion: spring ligament), tibiocal-caneal (origin: intercollicular groove-insertion: sustenaculum

tali), superficial posterior tibiotalar (origin: intercollicular groove-insertion:post inferior medial talar body)(Campbell JBJS Am 96: e62(1-10).

- **Ankle-anterior:** Anterior inferior tibiofibular (Chaput tubercle anterior lateral tibia-Wagstaffe tubercle fibula), **posterior**-post inferior tibiofibular, transverse, **deep**-interosseous
- **Rearfoot: Spring ligament complex** components: inferoplantar longitudinal, medioplantar oblique, superomedial (calcaneus—navicular) supports head of talus; **Subtalar joint lateral:** superficial (lateral talocalc, calcfib, lateral root inferior extensor retinaculum), intermediate (cervical, intermediate root inferior ext retinaculum), deep (interosseous talocalcaneal, medial root inferior extensor retinaculum) (*Core Knowledge in Orthopaedics-DiGiovanni CW*, 2007, p. 227); **bifurcate**-calcaneocuboid, calcaneonavicular, **cervical**-talocalcaneal, **long plantar**-calcaneus to cuboid and metatarsal base (limits midtarsal joint pronation), **short plantar**-calcaneal cuboid (limits midtarsal joint pronation)
- **Midfoot/Forefoot: Lisfranc-medial cuneiform** lateral surface to **2nd metatarsal** medial base; intermetatarsal ligaments at base of metatarsals except no ligament between 1st and 2nd metatarsal bases; TMT ligaments-stronger plantar than dorsal; cuneonavicular, cubonavicular, intercuneiform; deep transverse intermetatarsal connects adjacent plantar plates under the metatarsal (enhances stability of MTP joints) heads; collateral (MTP and IP joints, dorsal proximal to plantar distal), metatarsosesamoid, phalangeal sesamoid, interosseous sesamoids , Proper collateral ligament: metatarsal head tubercle->distal plantar->attach base proximal phalanx, Accessory collateral ligament: metatarsal head tubercle->plantar-> plantar plate

PLANTAR PLATE

- Fibrocartilaginous; attachments: Proximal-plantar fascia, plantar metatarsal neck, flexor tendon sheath, distal-plantar base proximal phalanx, medial/lateral-deep transverse intermetatarsal ligament, collateral ligaments attach to met head
- **Function:** Distal attachment of plantar fascia enabling windlass mechanism, fibrocartilage supports compressive loads, major stabilizer of lesser MTP joints (FAI 16:480-486)

PLANTAR FASCIA (APONEUROSIS)

- **Central band:** Origin-medial calcaneal tubercle, adheres to FDB, receives fibers from Achilles, plantaris; under midshaft of metatarsals divides into five superficial longitudinal tracts, proximal to met heads forms septate; insertion-deep (plantar plate, transverse metatarsal ligament, flexor sheath), superficial (subcutaneous, skin around MTP joints, base proximal phalanges), width 1.5 to 2 cm; medial band, lateral band, stabilizes arch via the windless mechanism

RETINACULUM

- **Fibular (peroneal): Superior**—attaches post lateral ridge of lateral malleolus to lateral calcaneus, **inferior**-inferior extensor retinaculum to lateral calcaneus (with attachment to the peroneal trochlea), covers fibularis (peroneus) brevis and longus
- **Flexor:** Attaches medial malleolus to medial calcaneus tuberosity; covers-1st compartment-tibialis post, 2nd-FDL, 3rd-post tib artery, venae comitantes, post tibial nerve, 4th-FHL
- **Extensor: Superior**—attaches inferior tibia and anterior fibular, **inferior**—attaches lateral calcaneus via upper stem to medial malleolus, and lower stem to plantar aponeurosis. Overlies (medial→lateral) tibialis anterior, EHL, anterior tibial artery, venae comitantes, deep fibular (peroneal) nerve, EDL, peroneus tertius

FOOT PLANTAR COMPARTMENTS

Nine compartments (FAI 10:267-275)
- **Medial:** Abductor hallucis, FHB
- **Superficial:** FDB, lumbricals, FDL tendon
- **Lateral:** Abductor digiti minimi, flexor digiti minimi
- **Adductor:** Adductor hallucis
- **Interosseous** (four compartments)
- **Calcaneal:** Quadratus plantae
- **Skin compartment** identified (Clinical Anatomy 20:201-208)
- **Calcaneal compartment:** not confirmed (JBJS Br 83-B: 245-249)

BURSA

- Retro Achilles, retrocalcaneus, plantar calcaneus, medial and lateral malleolus, insertion of tendons of tib anterior and tib post, intermetatarsophalangeal

OTHER

- **Synovial tendon sheath:** Tibialis anterior, EHL, EDL, EDB, fibularis (peroneus) longus, fibularis (peroneus) brevis, tibialis posterior, FHL, FDL
- **Heel fat pad:** Spiral septae of fibrous compartments containing columns of adipose tissue
- **Kager triangle:** Borders: inferior-superior surface of calcaneus, posterior-Achilles, anterior-FHL tendon

ARTERIES

- **Anterior tibial:** Tibial recurrent-anterior and post, anterior malleolar-medial and lateral, muscular, perforating, distal to ankle joint-dorsalis pedis
- **Posterior tibial:** Peroneal (posterior lateral malleolar, lateral calcaneal, fibula nutrient), medial malleolar, calcaneal, medial plantar, lateral plantar, tibial nutrient, circumflex fibularis
  Medial plantar: Digital branches anastomose with plantar metatarsal arteries
  Lateral plantar: Plantar arch → 1,2,3,4 plantar metatarsal arteries → plantar digital, perforating
- **Dorsalis pedis: Medial tarsal, lateral tarsal, 1st dorsal metatarsal → deep plantar**, dorsal digital; **arcuate →** 2nd, 3rd, 4th dorsal metatarsal → perforating, dorsal digital
- **Angiosomes:** Heel-post tib, peroneal; plantar foot-post tib; dorsal-anterior tib; lateral heel-peroneal, Hallux-dorsal and plantar angiosomes; medial ankle-anterior tib, lateral ankle-peroneal, anterior tib
- **Blood supply 1st metatarsal:** Nutrient A: penetrates lateral diaphysis, usually 1st dorsal met A, prox and distal br anastomose nck, head A; Periosteal A: 1st dorsal and plantar met A, sup br medial plantar A; Metaphyseal-Capital A: dorsal metaphyseal (dorsal 2/3 head), plantar metaphyseal (plantar 1/3 head), capital (medial, lateral 1/4 head) (*FAI* 8:81-93)

VEINS

- **Superficial:** Dorsal digital → metatarsal → venous arch →
  - **Medial marginal** → greater saphenous (anterior to medial malleolus)
  - **Lateral marginal** → lesser saphenous (posterior to lateral malleolus)
- **Deep veins:** Accompany arteries

LYMPH

- **Lymph** drains from foot primarily into **inguinal nodes** although some drain into popliteal nodes

NERVES

- **Tibial:**
  - **Sural** (posterior to lateral malleolus) → lateral dorsal cutaneous → dorsal digital lateral 5th toe
  - **Muscular:** FDL, FHL, TP, gastrocsoleus, plantaris, popliteus-soleus, popliteus
  - **Medial calcaneal**
  - **Medial plantar** → 1st, 2nd, 3rd common plantar → proper plantar to 1st, 2nd, 3rd digital cleft, proper to hallux Muscular to: abductor hallucis, FHB, 1st lumbrical, FDB
  - **Lateral plantar** → **superficial**-4th common plantar digital → proper digital to 4th cleft
    Muscular: Flex dig min brevis, 3rd plantar interosseous, 4th dorsal interossei quadratus plantae, abductor digiti minimi (quinti)
  - → **Deep**-muscular: add halluces; 2nd, 3rd, 4th lumbricals; 1st, 2nd, 3rd dorsal interossei; 1st, 2nd plantar interosei
  - **Common fibular(peroneal): Superficial** → **medial:** cutaneous-dorsal digital medial hallux, cutaneous cleft 2 and **intermediate**-dorsal cutaneous cleft 3, 4, Muscular → peroneus longus and brevis;
    Deep → **muscular**-tib anterior, EHL, EDL, peroneus tertius
    Medial terminal → cutaneous-1st dorsal digital cleft.
    Lateral terminal → muscular—EDB
  - **Saphenous:** Branch of femoral nerve (only nerve in foot that does not originate from sciatic), anterior to medial malleolus, **cutaneous**—medial ankle and foot (may extend to great toe)
  - **Baxter:** 1st branch of lateral plantar nerve, motor to abductor digiti minimi

Cutaneous Nerves

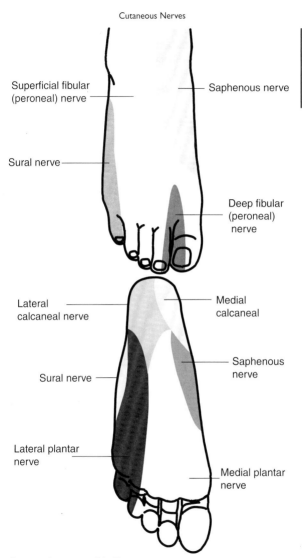

Superficial fibular (peroneal) nerve

Saphenous nerve

Sural nerve

Deep fibular (peroneal) nerve

Lateral calcaneal nerve

Medial calcaneal

Sural nerve

Saphenous nerve

Lateral plantar nerve

Medial plantar nerve

Cutaneous Innervation of the Foot

DERMATOMES

- **S1**-plantar heel and lateral foot (weak plantarflexion, decrease ankle reflex), **L5**-central plantar and dorsal foot (foot drop), **L4**-medial foot and medial ankle (foot drop) Figure-Dermatomes

Dermatomes

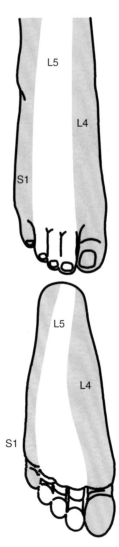

OTHER BONES

- **Accessory bones:** Os tibiale: navicular tuberosity, os trigonum: talus posterolateral tubercle
- **Sesamoids:** Constant-1st MTP joint, common sub-hallux IP joint, os peroneum (peroneus longus tendon)

COALITION

- **Talocalcaneal:** Subtalar joint middle facet, **calcaneonavicular**
- **Types:** Syndesmosis (fibrous), synchondrosis (cartilaginous), synostosis (osseous)

SURFACE LANDMARKS

- Medial malleolus, lateral malleolus, ankle joint, talonavicular joint, calcaneal cuboid joint, TMT joint, MTP joints, IP joints, navicular and 5th metatarsal tuberosity, metatarsal heads, sesamoids, sinus tarsus, tib anterior, EHL, EDL, peroneals, tib post, FDL, FHL, Achilles, EDB, dorsalis pedis, post tib artery, calcaneal tuberosity, talar head

Common locations of symptoms / signs of foot disorders

Dorsal

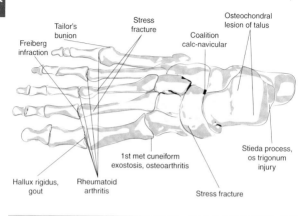

Tailor's bunion

Stress fracture

Freiberg infraction

Coalition calc-navicular

Osteochondral lesion of talus

1st met cuneiform exostosis, osteoarthritis

Hallux rigidus, gout

Rheumatoid arthritis

Stress fracture

Stieda process, os trigonum injury

Plantar

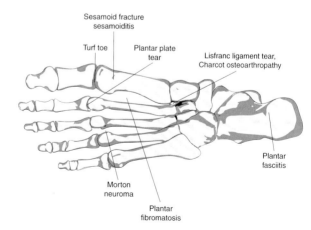

Sesamoid fracture sesamoiditis

Turf toe

Plantar plate tear

Lisfranc ligament tear, Charcot osteoarthropathy

Plantar fasciitis

Morton neuroma

Plantar fibromatosis

Medial

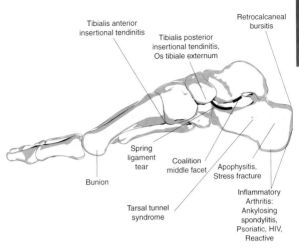

Tibialis anterior insertional tendinitis

Tibialis posterior insertional tendinitis, Os tibiale externum

Retrocalcaneal bursitis

Bunion

Spring ligament tear

Coalition middle facet

Apophysitis, Stress fracture

Tarsal tunnel syndrome

Inflammatory Arthritis: Ankylosing spondylitis, Psoriatic, HIV, Reactive

Lateral

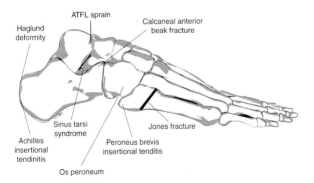

Haglund deformity

ATFL sprain

Calcaneal anterior beak fracture

Achilles insertional tendinitis

Sinus tarsi syndrome

Peroneus brevis insertional tenditis

Jones fracture

Os peroneum

BIOMECHANICS AND GAIT

EDWARD LEE • WINSTON L. TROPE • ROCK C. J. POSITANO • ROCK G. POSITANO • RONALD M. GUBERMAN

CARDINAL BODY PLANES

- **Frontal or coronal:** Bisects body into front and back. Motion = Flexion/extension
- **Sagittal:** Bisects body into left and right. Motion = Abduction/adduction
- **Transverse:** Bisects body into superior and inferior halves. Motion = Internal/external rotation

BIOMECHANICAL ASSESSMENT

- Weight-bearing assessment in **angle and base of gait**
- **Angle of gait:** Degree of abduction from midsagittal plane. Normal = 7° to 10° abducted
- **Base of gait:** Distance between medial malleoli. Normal = 8 to 10 cm
- Assess muscle strength, ROM, position of hip, knee, ankle, midtarsal, subtalar, 1st ray, 1st MPJ, digits
- **Relaxed calcaneal stance position:** Angular deviation between bisection of heel and perpendicular line from ground
- **Neutral calcaneal stance position:** With subtalar joint (STJ) in **neutral**, the angular deviation between bisection of heel and perpendicular line from ground
- **Structural limb length:** Anatomic length of femur and tibia. Measured from anterior superior iliac spine (**ASIS**) to **medial/lateral malleolus**
- **Functional limb length:** Lengths of limb when weight bearing or ambulating. Anatomic lengths equal, but limb discrepancy caused by spinal abnormality, asymmetric knee, ankle, or rearfoot alignment, or muscle contractures. Measured from **umbilicus** to **medial/lateral malleolus** (*The PI Manual*, Podiatry Institute, 1999)

COMBINED LIMB LENGTH DISCREPANCY

- Asymmetrical limb length causes significantly **increased loading and stress** on the joints of the lower back, particularly on the side of the longer limb.
- The greater the discrepancy, the greater the abnormal loading

- Two main forms and one minor form of limb length discrepancy (LLD): Structural (main), functional (main), environmental (minor)
  - **Structural:** Anatomic LLD, such as shortened **malformation** of one or more bones in the leg or ankle. May be caused by epiphyseal injury, unequal development, fracture with shortening or lengthening, sacral deformities, innominate deformities, or arthritis. Manifests as pelvic obliquity with anterior and posterior superior iliac spines low on the same side, leveled by a heel lift
  - **Functional:** LLD due to **joint contracture** or **axial misalignments**. May be caused by pelvic obliquity, adduction contracture or flexion contracture of the hip, genu varum, valgum, or recurvatum, calcaneovalgus, equinovarus, or rearfoot pronation. When secondary to foot pronation, manifests as pelvic obliquity, with anterior and posterior superior iliac spines low on the same side, and is leveled by supinating the STJ to a neutral position
  - **Environmental:** LLD from **extracorporeal, environmental factors** such as movement surface or footwear
- **Limb length asymmetry compensation**: Comorbidities of LLD include scoliosis, lower back pain, knee and/or hip arthritis, plantar fasciitis, medial tibial stress syndrome, Achilles tendonitis (shorter limb), and metatarsalgia. Below are the most common presentations of LLD as noted by Beilke:
  - **Sacral and pelvic tilt toward the short limb**: The most common method of biomechanical compensation for LLD is the sacral spine's conforming to the tilt of the pelvis toward the shorter limb, resulting in convex lumbar curve toward the short side.
  - **Sacral and pelvic tilt toward the long limb without lumbar curve**: The sacrum overcompensates for the LLD and tilts toward the longer leg, making the sacrum almost level and removing the lumbar curve.
  - **Sacral tilt toward the long limb with lumbar curve**: Like the second type, the sacrum tilts toward the longer limb, but lumbar curve becomes convex toward the long side.
- In addition to standard methods of LLD testing, given below, patient's **gait** should also be analyzed to check for **midstride asymmetries**, which may be apparent in altered gait timing.
  - Diagnosis can be made using several methods, including **pelvic X-ray**, **Schwab test**, placing the fingers at the small

part of the iliac crests near the posterior superior spines and visually comparing, or **palpatory method**, checking iliac crests, greater femoral trochanters, posterior and anterior iliac spines, inferior scapular tips, and acromioclavicular joints for differences in height.

- Clinicians should also note any pelvic side shift, lateral spine curvature and convexity, frontal, sagittal, and transverse planar leg deviation, or unilateral foot pronation.
- Differentiation of various functional LLDs can be made using the **Beekman pronation test.**
  - If pronation alters limb length, causes functional leg shortening, compensates for longer leg, or causes sacroiliac dysfunction
  - If pronation lowers superior iliac spine on ipsilateral side relative to neutral foot positioning, orthoses are indicated for a functional LLD.
  - If iliac spine is leveled by pronation of feet, heel lift is indicated on the side opposite leveling pronation.
  - If pronation decreases ASIS and increases ipsilateral posterior superior iliac spine, orthoses are indicated to resolve asymmetric pelvic pronation.
- Alternatively, clinicians can utilize digital methods, such as **motion capture cameras**, **pressure or force plates**, or **eMed pads** to analyze patients' footstep and gait or ensure proper performance of pronation tests.
- Beware of the development of equinus deformity of the ankle in patients with an internal heel lift. Deformity development indicates an inadequate lift and the need for an additional, external lift.
- Using heel lifts and orthotics to compensate for length discrepancy and alter loading would correct biomechanical deficiency.
  - Baylis WJ, Rzonca EC. Functional and structural limb length discrepancies: evaluation and treatment. *Clin Podiatr Med Surg.* 1988;5(3):509-520.
  - Kiapour A, Abdelgawad AA, Goel VK, Souccar A, Terai T, Ebraheim NA. Relationship between limb length discrepancy and load distribution across the sacroiliac joint—a finite element study. *J Orthop Res.* 2012;30(10):1577-1580. doi:10.1002/jor.22119.

Limb Length Discrepancy Type (LLD)			
	Structural (Major)	**Functional (Major)**	**Environmental (Minor)**
Nature of discrepancy	Anatomic, such as shortening of a long bone	Effective, such as joint shortening or axial misalignments	Imposed by environment, such as movement surface or footwear
Possible causes	Epiphyseal injury, unequal development, fracture with shortening or lengthening, sacral deformities, innominate deformities, or arthritis	Pelvic obliquity, adduction contracture or flexion contracture of the hip, genu varum, valgum, or recurvatum, calcaneovalgus, equinovarus, or rearfoot pronation	Movement surface or footwear

Normal Joint Range of Motion (NWB)		
Joint	**Normal Range**	**Notes**
Hip		
Rotation	45° internal and external	1:1 internal:external rotation
Flexion	90°-100° (w/knee extended) 120°-130° (w/knee flexed)	–
Extension	10°-20°	–
ABduction/ ADduction	24°-60°/<30°	–
Knee		
Flexion/extension	130°-150°/5°-10°	>10° extensions = Genu Recurvatum
Rotation	40° internal and external	–
Patellar position	Midline	Line up with 2nd digit/ metatarsal

Normal Joint Range of Motion (NWB) (continued)		
Joint	**Normal Range**	**Notes**
Ankle		
Dorsiflexion/plantarflexion	10°-20°/20°-40°	**Silverskiold test**; <10° DF w/knee extended or <20° DF w/knee flexed = Equinus
Malleolar position	13°-18° externally rotated	–
Midtarsal		**Transverse:frontal:sagittal**
Oblique axis	DF/PF, AD/ABduction	**52°:38°:57°**
Longitudinal axis	Inversion/eversion	15°:**75°**:9°
Subtalar	20° inversion:10° eversion 2:1 inversion:eversion	42° from sagittal, 16° from transverse Triplanar motion
1st Ray (DF/PF)	±5 mm	–
1st MPJ	65°-75° dorsiflexion	–

POSTURAL ASSESSMENT

- **Head:** Centered from lateral view, midline of body from AP view. No tilting left/right during gait.
- **Shoulder:** Level and even. No tilting/dropping during gait.
- **Pelvis:** Level. ASIS even. No excessive tilting/dropping during gait.
- **Arm swing:** Moderate and even swing during gait.

GAIT

- Gait = **2 Phases**, stance (62%) and swing (38%)
- Stance phase further divided into **three periods**: Contact, midstance, propulsive
- **Gait cycle:** Measured from heel contact of one foot to heel contact of the same foot.
- **Step length:** Distance between heel contact of one foot to the contralateral foot.
- **Stride length:** Distance between successive heel contacts of the same foot. Stride length = 2 × step length.
- **Cadence:** Speed of gait = steps per minute.
- **Double limb support:** Portion of gait cycle when both feet are in contact with the ground. Accounts for **25%** of gait. *****No double support when running**.
- **Float:** Period during running when no limb is in contact with the ground.

***This is a key feature of gait that is missing when a patient is running.

	Stance phase			
Heel strike	Foot flat	Heel rise	Push-off	Toe-off
0%	15%	30%	45%	60%

	Swing phase		
Acceleration	Toe clearance	Deceleration	Heel strike
70%	85%	100%	

Nordin M, Frankel VH. *Basic Biomechanics of the Musculoskeletal System.* Philadelphia, PA: Wolters Kluwer Health/Lippincott Williams & Wilkins; 2012.

STJ MOTION DURING GAIT

- At heel strike, STJ starts pronation for shock absorption →
  Supinates during midstance, locking midtarsal joint → Locked
  midtarsal joint creates rigid lever arm in medial column →
  forefoot weight shifts from lateral to medial → Propulsion
  and toe-off

GAIT PATTERNS

Gait Pattern	Description	Associated Disorders	Notes
Antalgic	Decreased weight-bearing duration on painful limb, resulting in a limp	Osteoarthritis, foot/ankle sprains, fractures, metatarsalgia, neuroma	–
Hemiplegic (spastic)	Broad-based, unilateral; Affected limb in extension and foot plantarflexed; ↓ stance phase on affected side and affected limb circumduction in swing	Stroke	Tonus of upper limb flexor muscles, arm close to body
Diplegic (scissoring)	Narrow base; dragging of bilateral limbs and toes. Slightly flexed knee and hips in adducted position. **Circumduction** of both limbs in swing	Cerebral palsy, Parkinson	–
Coxalgic	Upper trunk shifted toward painful side without pelvic tilt during stance phase	Disorders associated with hip pain	–
Waddling	Broad-based, dropping of swinging limb; pelvic drops on contralateral side because of weakness of **gluteus medius** (Trendelenburg sign)	Muscular dystrophy	–

(continued)

Gait Pattern	Description	Associated Disorders	Notes
Steppage	Weak extensors causing affected limb to be lifted higher during swing phase. Results in **slapping of foot** on contact.	Peroneal nerve palsy, L5 radiculopathy, CMT	**Drop foot**; Unable to stand on heels or perform toe walking
Cerebellar ataxia	Broad-based, irregular, and variable stride length. Clumsy, staggering. Upper body swaying (**Titubation**)	Cerebellar lesions	Unable to perform **tandem walking**; resembles alcohol intoxicated gait
Sensory ataxia	Broad-based, irregular and variable stride length	Polyneuropathy, dorsal column lesions	Unable to perform **Romberg test** (walking with eye's closed). Gait worsens without visual input
Shuffling	Narrow base, stooped neck, shoulder, and trunk posture. Feet lifted minimally above ground during swing. ↓Stride length↑cadence	Parkinson	**Festination** (↓stride length↑cadence)
Choreatic	Broad-based and slow. Irregular, **dance-like**, involuntary, jerking. Variable stride length and direction	Huntington	–

Wien Klin Wochenschr 2017;129:81; Gait Abnormalities | Stanford Medicine 25 | Stanford Medicine. Web. 30 April, 2017.

Links Between the Lower Extremities and Axial Skeleton

- Posture of the foot and ankle has direct consequences for spinal health.
- Excessive pronation of the STJ results in overuse injuries.
- Excessive STJ pronation also leads to internal rotation of the tibia and femur, tilting the pelvis anteriorly, and increasing loading and strain on the sacral and lumbar spines.
- Pronated pedal posture has strong correlation with lower back pain in women.
- Prescription orthoses and gait alteration are viable therapies for resolution of lower back pain in individuals with biomechanical aberrations in their feet and ankles.

Suggested Readings

Kendall JC, Bird AR, Azari MF. Foot posture, leg length discrepancy and low back pain—their relationship and clinical management using foot orthoses—an overview. *Foot.* 2014;24(2):75-80. doi:10.1016/j.foot.2014.03.004.

Khamis S, Yizhar Z. Effect of feet hyperpronation on pelvic alignment in a standing position. *Gait Posture.* 2007;25(1):127-134. doi:10.1016/j.gaitpost.2006.02.005.

Menz HB, Dufour AB, Riskowski JL, Hillstrom HJ, Hannan MT. Foot Posture, foot function and low back pain: the Framingham Foot Study. *Rheumatology.* 2013;52(12):2275-2282. doi:10.1093/rheumatology/ket298.

RADIOLOGY AND IMAGING I

RONALD M. GUBERMAN

TERMINOLOGY

- **Orthoposer:** Platform designed to take weight-bearing X-rays. Often attached to the tubehead with a fixed arm
- **Tubehead:** Lead-lined and oil-filled housing for the X-ray tube. The tubehead is manipulated to aim and direct the X-ray beam.
- **Cassette:** Rigid film/screen holders placed between the patient and tubehead against the anatomic area of interest that receives the X-ray beam
- **Kilovoltage (kVp):** Determines speed of electrons emitted. Affects the frequency and wavelength of the emitted electrons. ↑kVp, ↓contrast and vice versa
- **Milliamperage (MaS):** Determines number of electrons emitted. Product of milliampere multiplied by exposure time. ↑MaS, ↑density and vice versa.
- **Rad:** Unit of absorbed radiation dose
- **Roentgen:** Unit of exposed radiation (Christman RA. *Foot Ankle Radiol* 2003)
- **Roentgen equivalent man (rem):** Amount of ionizing radiation absorbed by humans to produce a biologic effect (ie, radiation-induced cancer):
  - 1 rem = 1 Sievert (same measurement, different unit; more commonly used SI unit outside of the United States),
  - 1 rem = 0.055% of developing cancer,
  - Maximum permissible dose = **5 rem/year.**

ELEMENTS OF EXPOSURE

- **Focal spot:** Smaller the focal spot, better the image.
- **Exposure time:** Increased exposure time increases amount of electrons emitted. Increasing exposure time increases image density.
- **Density:** The whiteness and blackness of an image. Dependent on amount of photons emitted, controlled by milliamperage and exposure time
  ↑MaS, ↑density and vice versa
  Contrast: The difference in densities between structures. Allows for increase in detail and visualization of adjacent structures. Controlled by kilovolts. ↑kVp, ↓contrast and vice versa.

- **Distance:** Affects density of image. Greater the distance, the fewer photons strike film, which decreases density.
  Inverse square law: As distance is increased by a factor x, the amount of photons striking the film decreases by $1/x^2$ (Christman RA. *Foot Ankle Radiol* 2003).
  Example: If distance is doubled, $1/2^2$ or $1/4$ of emitted photons strike film. If tripled, $1/3^2$ or $1/9$ of emitted photons strike film.

PRINCIPLES OF X-RAYS

- **Primary radiation:** Radiation exposure from the X-ray beam directly emitted from the tubehead
- **Secondary radiation:** Radiation exposure after the X-ray beam has passed through the target
- **Compton effect:** Scatter radiation caused by interaction between incoming photon and outer shell electron
- **Photoelectric effect:** Absorbed radiation caused by interaction between incoming photon and inner shell electron
- **Hard X-ray:** Radiographs created with high kVp. ↑kVp, ↓wavelength, ↑frequency, ↑penetration. Safer for patient because of ↓radiation absorption
- **Soft X-ray:** Radiographs created with low kVp. ↓kVp, ↑wavelength, ↓frequency, ↓penetration. More harmful to patient because of ↑radiation absorption (Christman RA. *Foot Ankle Radiol* 2003)
- **Radiographic Views and Angles:** Tables 1-1 to 1-3

OTTAWA RULES

- Rules to access when foot or ankle radiographs are necessary after an acute injury
- Ankle X-rays necessary if pain in the malleolar zone plus 1 of the following:
  - Tenderness along distal 6 mm posterior edge of tibia or tip of medial malleolus **OR**
  - Tenderness along distal 6 mm posterior edge of fibula or tip of lateral malleolus **OR**
  - Unable to weight bear for four steps
- Foot X-rays necessary if pain in the midfoot zone plus 1 of the following (*JAMA* 1993;269(9):1127):
  - Tenderness at base of 5th metatarsal **OR**
  - Tenderness at navicular **OR**
  - Unable to weight bear for four steps

TABLE 1-1 Radiographic Foot Views				
Foot X-ray View	Position of Foot	Position of Tubehead	Aim of Central Ray	Notes
AP or DP	Flat, angle, and base of gait	15° from vertical	2nd metatarsocuneiform joint	–
Lateral	Medial aspect against plate	90° from vertical	5th metatarsal-cuboid joint	–
Medial oblique (WB)	Flat	45° from vertical, lateral side	4th metatarsal-cuboid joint	Visualize CN bar
Medial oblique (NWB)	45° with medial aspect of foot against cassette	0° from vertical	3rd metatarsocuneiform joint	Visualize CN bar
Lateral oblique (WB)	Flat	45° from vertical, medial side	1st metatarsocuneiform joint	–
Lateral oblique (NWB)	45° with lateral aspect of foot against cassette	0° from vertical	1st metatarsocuneiform joint	–
Sesamoid axial	Toes pointed toward cassette, hallux dorsiflexed, heel slightly elevated	90° from vertical, posterior	Plantar surface of 3rd metatarsal head	Visualize sesamoidal fractures
Calcaneal axial	Flat, leaning slightly forward	45° from vertical, posterior	In between insertion of Achilles tendon and ankle joint	Visualize calc body, middle/posterior facets of STJ

(continued)

TABLE 1-1 Radiographic Foot Views (continued)

Foot X-Ray View	Position of Foot	Position of Tubehead	Aim of Central Ray	Notes
Modified calcaneal axial	Flat, leaning slightly forward	0° from vertical	Posterior aspect of heel	Visualize posterior heel spurs
Harris-Beath (ski-jump)	Flat, bend knees	45° from vertical, posterior	Center of heel	Visualize talocalcaneal coalitions
Borden	Supine, heel against cassette, foot internally rotated 45°	10°, 20°, 30°, 40° from vertical	Between lateral malleoli and 5th metatarsal base	Visualize posterior facet of STJ
Isherwood—lateral oblique	Cassette medial, externally rotated 45°	0° from vertical	1 inch below and anterior to lateral malleoli	Visualize anterior facet of STJ
Isherwood—medial oblique axial	Cassette medial, foot dorsiflexed and inverted, externally rotated 30°	10° cephalad from vertical	1 inch below and anterior to lateral malleoli	Visualize middle facet of STJ
Isherwood—lateral oblique axial	Cassette lateral, foot dorsiflexed and everted, internally rotated 30°	10° cephalad from vertical	1 inch below medial malleoli	Visualize posterior facet of STJ
Canale	Flat, max equinus and pronated 15°	75° from horizontal (or 15° from vertical)	Talus	Visualize talar neck

Adapted from Christman RA. Foot Ankle Radiol, 2003; J Bone Joint Surg 1961;43B:566; J Bone Joint Surg Am 1978;60:143.

TABLE 1-2 Radiographic Ankle Views

Ankle X-ray View	Position	Position of Tubehead	Aim of Central Ray	Notes
AP	Heel against cassette, midline of foot perpendicular to cassette	90° from vertical	Center of ankle joint	–
Lateral	Medial aspect against cassette	90° from vertical	Center of ankle joint	–
Mortise	Internally rotated 15°	90° from vertical	Center of ankle joint	–
Medial oblique	Internally rotated 45°	90° from vertical	Center of ankle joint	–
Lateral oblique	Externally rotated 45°	90° from vertical	Center of ankle joint	–
Stressed inversion (talar tilt)	Same as AP; patient supine; invert heel	0° from vertical	Center of ankle joint	Evaluate ATFL/CFL; ≥5° compared with contralateral or >10° abnormal
Anterior drawer	Same as lateral; patient supine; pull heel anteriorly	0° from vertical	Center of ankle joint	Evaluate ATFL; >6 mm displacement suggestive of ATFL rupture

(continued)

TABLE 1-2 Radiographic Ankle Views (continued)

Ankle X-Ray View	Position	Position of Tubehead	Aim of Central Ray	Notes
External rotation	Same as Mortise; patient supine; externally rotate foot	0° from vertical	Center of ankle joint	Evaluate deltoid ligament; Medial clear space >4 mm and >1 mm than superior joint space suggestive of deltoid injury
Stressed plantarflexion	Same as lateral foot view; patient supine	0° from vertical	5th metatarsal-cuboid joint	AKA **Eyre-Brook View**; Calcaneovalgus vs vertical talus; If talus and 1st met align = Calcaneovalgus

Adapted from Christman RA. Foot Ankle Radiol, 2003; J Bone Joint Surg Am 2004;86:2171.

TABLE 1-3 Radiographic Angles

Angle	View	Description	Normal Values	Notes
Intermetatarsal angle (IM)	AP view	Bisection of 1st and 2nd metatarsals	8°-12°	–
Metatarsus adductus angle (MA)	AP view	Bisection of 2nd met to perpendicular bisection of tarsal bones	0°-15°	MA angle >15° added to IM to calculate **true IM**
Hallux abductus angle	AP view	Bisection of proximal phalanx and 1st metatarsal	10°-20°	–
Hallux Interphalangeal angle	AP view	Bisection of distal and proximal phalanx	0°-10°	

	TABLE 1-3 Radiographic Angles (*continued*)			
Angle	**View**	**Description**	**Normal Values**	**Notes**
Proximal articular set angle	AP view	Perpendicular line to bisection of 1st met to effective articular cartilage of 1st met head	0°-8°	–
Distal articular set angle	AP view	Bisection of proximal phalanx to effective articular cartilage of proximal phalanx base	0°-8°	–
Tibial sesamoid position	AP view	Position of tibial sesamoid relative to 1st metatarsal	Positions 1-3	Position 1 (medial); Position 7 (lateral); Position 4 = midpoint
4th/5th intermetatarsal angle	AP view	Bisection of 4th and 5th metatarsals	8°-10°	Can also be measured by bisection to 5th met to medial border of 5th met (**Fallat and Buckholz**)
Lateral deviation	AP view	Bisection of 5th met head and medial border of 5th met	0°-8°	–
Metatarsal protrusion	AP view	Difference between distal distance of 1st and 2nd mets	±2 mm	–

(*continued*)

TABLE 1-3 Radiographic Angles (*continued*)

Angle	View	Description	Normal Values	Notes
Kite angle	AP view	Bisection of talus and calcaneus	15°-35°	–
Cuboid abduction angle	AP view	Lateral borders of cuboid and calcaneus	0°-5°	Increased in flatfoot
Calcaneal inclination angle	Lateral view	Plantar border of calcaneus to ground	18°-21°	Increased in cavus, decreased in flatfoot
Meary angle	Lateral view	Bisection of 1st met and Talus	0°-5°	–
Cyma line	Lateral view	Smooth S-curve formed by TN and CC joint	Smooth, continuous S-curve	Talus anterior break = Pronation Calcaneal anterior break = Supination
Böhler angle	Lateral view	Posterosuperior border of calcaneal body to line created by superior points of anterior process and posterior facet	20°-40°	Decreased in calcaneal fractures
Gissane angle	Lateral view	Borders of posterior and anterior/middle facet	120°-140°	Increased in calcaneal fractures
Fowler-Philip angle	Lateral view	Posterior and plantar borders of calcaneus	44°-69°	>75° = Pathologic

TABLE 1-3 Radiographic Angles (*continued*)				
Angle	View	Description	Normal Values	Notes
Total angle	Lateral view	Calcaneal inclination + Fowler-Philip	90°	>90° suggestive of Haglund deformity
Angle of hibbs	Lateral view	Bisection of 1st met to plantar border of calcaneus	>150°	<150° suggestive of cavus

Adapted from *McGlamry's Comprehensive Textbook of Foot and Ankle Surgery.* 4th ed. LWW.

OTHER IMAGING MODALITIES

- **Ultrasound:** Use of high frequency sound waves. **Nonionizing radiation**. White = Hyper**echoic**, Black = Hypo**echoic**. Primarily used to assess soft tissue pathology. Good for foreign bodies, plantar fasciitis, Achilles tendon pathology, neuromas, soft tissue masses, plantar plate pathology, ankle ligaments.
- **Computerized tomography:** Multiple X-rays from various angles compiled by computer. Primarily used to visualize osseous and soft tissue pathology. **Cartilage not visualized**. Good for osseous pathologies involving cortical bone (ie, fractures). Contrast may be used to enhance image.
- **Magnetic resonance imaging (MRI):** Use of low energy radio frequencies produced by a magnetic field. **Nonionizing radiation**. Primarily used to visualize osseous and soft tissue pathology. T1 versus T2-weighted MRIs. Contrast may be used to enhance soft tissue image.
- **T1-weighted MRI:** Anatomic. Short TR and TE. **Fat** dependent, fat displayed with highest signal intensity
- **T2-weighted MRI:** Pathologic. Long TR and TE. **Water** dependent, water displayed with highest signal intensity, suggestive of inflammation
- **Short T1 inversion MRI:** Fat suppressed using short TR. May be used with T1 or T2. Better visualization of soft tissue and pathology that may be hidden within fat. Decreases image artifacts
- **Gadolinium:** Injectable contrast medium for MRI/MRA for enhanced visualization of blood vessels and some tumors. Mechanism: shortens T1 relaxation time of protons.

- **Technetium-99m MDP (Tc-99m):** Tc-99m **M**ethylene **D**i-**P**hosphonate most commonly used. Labels hydroxyapatite crystals in bone. Renally excreted. Highly sensitive but nonspecific. Primarily used to visualize areas of **increased osteoblastic activity.** Any area of bony turnover, caused by physical stress, repair, or tumor, presents as "hot spots." Four phase scans available.
  - **Phase 1 (blood flow):** Immediate, within **seconds** of injection. Angiogram
  - **Phase 2 (blood pool):** 10 to 20 **minutes** after injection. Localized accumulation of isotope
  - **Phase 3 (delayed):** 2 to 4 **hours** after injection. Osseous uptake of isotope
  - **Phase 4 (24 hours):** 24 **hours** after injection. Isotope uptake stops at 4 hours in normal bone, but continues for 24 hours in pathologic bone. Also, useful in patients with decreased vascularity **(Table 1-4)**
- **Gallium-67 citrate (Ga-67):** Binds to leukocytes, lactoferrin, and transferrin. Images taken 24 hours after injection. Uptake of Ga-67 to localized areas of infection. Coupled with Tc-99m scan to rule out osteomyelitis
- **Indium-111 (In-111, Serotec):** Blood drawn from patient, patient's own WBC isolated and tagged with indium. Images taken 24 hours after injection. Uptake localized to areas of infection (Christman RA, *Foot and Ankle Radiology*, 2003; *The PI Manual*, Podiatry Institute, 1999)

TABLE 1-4 Bone Scan Results, Cellulitis Versus Osteomyelitis Versus Charcot

Bone Scan	Cellulitis	Osteomyelitis	Charcot
Tc-99m MDP	+	+	±
Tc-99m (Phase 1)	+++	+	±
Tc-99m (Phase 2)	++	++	±
Tc-99m (Phase 3)	+	+++	+++
Tc-99m (Phase 4)	−	+++	+++
Ga-67	+ (diffusely to ST)	+ (localized to bone)	−
In-111	+ (in ST)	+ (in bone)	−

The PI Manual, Podiatry Institute, 1999.

YOSHIMI ENDO

IMAGING MODALITIES USED FOR ASSESSING THE FOOT AND ANKLE

Table 1-1 Most common imaging modalities used for the foot and ankle with their advantages and disadvantages.

	Advantages	Disadvantages
X-ray	• Readily available • Cheap • With weight bearing, most accurate for assessing alignment	• Uses ionizing radiation • Poor soft tissue evaluation
Bone scan	• Good screening test • Very sensitive	• Uses ionizing radiation • Poor anatomic detail, thus not specific
Computed tomography (CT)	• Best study for bony/cortical detail • Some soft tissue detail	• Uses ionizing radiation
Magnetic resonance imaging (MRI)	• No ionizing radiation • Exquisite soft tissue detail • Also bony trabecular detail • Only modality to directly assess cartilage	• Not readily available • Expensive • Long acquisition time • Real contraindications • Certain materials can create debilitating artifact
Ultrasound (US)	• No ionizing radiation • Quick exam • Exquisite soft tissue detail • Can image even in the presence of metal • Allows dynamic maneuvers • Doppler for assessing vascularity and disease activity • Can use for image-guided procedures	• Operator dependent • Not readily available • Cannot evaluate through bone

Radiography (X-ray)

- **Routine ankle views:** AP, mortise, lateral
  Routine foot views: AP, oblique, lateral
  Additional views: Saltzman view, tangential (sesamoid) view
  (Fig. 1-1), Harris view, stress views

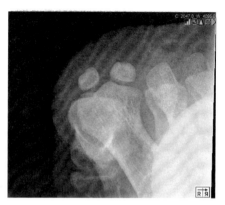

Figure 1-1 Normal sesamoid view radiograph of the foot.

- Most important initial modality in most clinical situations. Identifies fractures, bone tumors, and arthritides. When obtained weight bearing, can assess alignment. Soft tissue swelling can be identified on X-rays and may localize the site of injury.

Bone Scintigraphy (Bone Scan)

- Radioactive tracer (methylene diphosphonate [MDP]) labeled with technetium-99m (^{99m}**Tc MDP**) is injected into the patient intravenously. Distribution of the tracer can be recorded using a gamma camera. The skeletal phase, obtained after 2 to 4 hours, shows ↑ tracer uptake at sites of increased osteoblastic activity, including metastatic disease, fractures, arthritis, and osteomyelitis. Imaging at early phases, such as the flow phase at 5 seconds after injection and blood pool phase at 5 minutes after injection, can help narrow the DDx.
- The findings are often nonspecific but can be very useful in certain clinical scenarios because of the high sensitivity of the test.

Computed Tomography

- Multidetector row scanners allow sub-millimeter high spatial resolution and postprocessing to generate images in any plane.

- Cross-sectional evaluation is especially useful for diagnosing and characterizing fractures.
- Outstanding bone detail is ideal for assessing the degree of healing of fractures or osteotomies.
- "Windowing" the images facilitates evaluation of the soft tissues.

Magnetic Resonance Imaging
- Makes use of the fact that protons in different tissue environments become excited by an external magnetic field to different degrees.
- Exact set of pulse sequences acquired for each study varies based on institution and the body part, but typically consists of a combination of **T1W**, **T2W**, **PD** (proton density), and fat-saturated pulse sequences (eg, inversion recovery [**STIR**]) in various planes.
- Superb spatial resolution and soft tissue contrast make it an optimal modality for evaluating most pathologies in the foot and ankle.
- Although the field-of-view can be widened to include the entire foot and ankle in one exam, MRI exams should be focused to a specific region (ie, ankle/hindfoot, midfoot, or forefoot) to provide high-resolution, diagnostic-quality images.

Ultrasound
- Sound waves reflect at tissue interfaces, and the reflection is sensed by the US transducer and helps generate an image.
- Provides exquisite soft tissue detail for structures that are relatively superficial, such as tendons and ligaments of the foot and ankle, although US cannot assess inside or behind bones as sound does not penetrate through bone.
- Capability for dynamic maneuvers, "sonopalpation," and US-guided interventions are additional advantages of US over other modalities.

TRAUMATIC/OVERUSE BONE INJURIES

Traumatic Fractures
- Although traumatic fractures can occur in any bone, characteristic fractures involving certain bones commonly occur, dictated by the mechanism of injury.
- Many fractures are easily visible on routine three-view X-rays of the foot and/or ankle.
- CT is much more sensitive for subtle fractures in certain areas of the foot/ankle (eg, Lisfranc fracture-dislocations [**Fig. 1-2A**]). CT may also be indicated to better define the fracture that is identified on an X-ray.

- MRI is more sensitive than CT for trabecular fractures or bone contusions: Fractures that do not involve the cortex **(Fig. 1-2B)**. Trabecular fracture line will be hypointense (↓signal intensity [SI]) in all pulse sequences surrounded by area of bone marrow edema (↑SI on STIR or fat-saturated T2W/PD sequences).
- US, although usually not the primary modality to image fractures, can diagnose fractures that extend to the cortex.

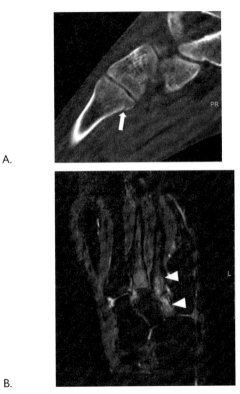

A.

B.

Figure 1-2 A, Sagittal reformation of a CT scan of the foot showing an acute nondisplaced fracture of the base of the 3rd metatarsal (arrow), which was occult on radiographs. B, MRI coronal IR sequence obtained on the same day shows trabecular fractures of the 2nd metatarsal and intermediate cuneiform (arrowheads), which were not visible on the CT scan in addition to the fracture of the 3rd metatarsal.

Stress Fractures

- Due to repetitive overuse, occur at characteristic locations in the foot and ankle, including the metatarsal shaft **(Fig. 1-3A)**, navicular **(Fig.1-3B)**, and posterior body of the calcaneus **(Fig.1-3C)**.
- May be radiographically occult for days to weeks. CT may also be insensitive. On X-ray and CT, stress fracture manifests as faint sclerosis, disruption of the cortex, and/or periosteal reaction.
- **MRI is very sensitive:** Stress reactions may manifest as focal bone marrow edema ± periosteal edema. Stress fractures

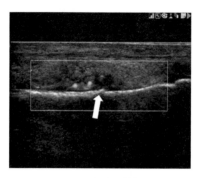

A.

B.

Figure 1-3 A, US long axis to the metatarsal shows cortical break and surrounding power Doppler hyperemia representing a stress fracture (arrow). B, CT with coronal reformation shows an acute navicular stress fracture (arrow). C, Lateral radiograph showing a calcaneal stress fracture (arrow).

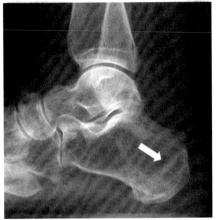

C.

Figure 1-3 (continued)

show a ↓SI line in the marrow oriented perpendicular to the long axis of the bone.

- Bone scan is very sensitive for even early stress fractures but lacks specificity **(Fig. 1-4)**.
- US is sensitive for stress fractures once there is cortical disruption. Earlier phase may be diagnosed using power Doppler to detect periosteal hyperemia.

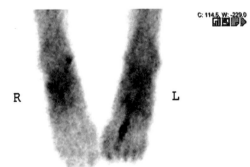

Figure 1-4 Delayed phase image of a three-phase bone scan showing focal uptake of the 2nd metatarsal shaft consistent with a stress fracture.

TENDONS

Normal Tendons

- CT allows a crude evaluation of tendons by "windowing" the images to optimize for soft tissues, but MRI and US are the most accurate modalities for assessing tendons.
- On MRI, tendons are homogeneously black on all pulse sequences and should remain uniform in shape and size throughout their course **(Fig. 1-5A)**. Mean AP thickness of the Achilles tendon is 5 to 6 mm (*Am J Roentgenol* 1999;173:323).
- Because all of the tendons of the foot and ankle are located relatively superficially, they are accurately evaluated on US. Normal tendons have a homogeneously hyperechoic (bright) fibrillary architecture that are of fixed thickness **(Fig. 1-5B)**.

Tendinosis

- Degenerative process of the tendon usually due to repetitive overuse.

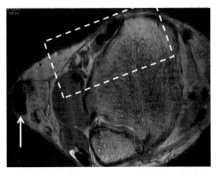

A.

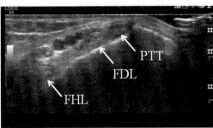

B.

Figure 1-5 A, Axial PD MRI shows normal tendons of the ankle, including the Achilles tendon (arrow). Dotted square indicates the region demonstrated in (B). B, US shows the flexor tendons in the tarsal tunnel.

- The tendon is thicker than normal (eg, >6 mm thick for the Achilles tendon) **(Fig. 1-6A)** with areas of abnormal ↑SI on MRI and areas that are heterogeneous and hypoechoic (dark) on US.

Tenosynovitis
- Inflammation of the tendon sheath, manifesting as fluid occupying the tendon sheath (↑SI on T2W/PD with or without fat saturation; hypoechoic layer of fluid surrounding the tendon on US ± hyperemia on Doppler).

Tendon Tear
- Discontinuity of fibers visible on both MRI and US. "Rupture" if complete discontinuity **(Fig. 1-6B)**. Longitudinal split tears most commonly occur in the peroneus brevis.
- Usually occurs in the background of chronic overuse, thus there will be an underlying tendinosis of the torn tendon with thickening and abnormal SI on MRI and areas of heterogeneity and ↓echogenicity on US.

LIGAMENTS

Normal Ligaments
- On MRI, normal ligaments are either a homogeneously black band of tissue on all pulse sequences (eg, Lisfranc ligament) or striated in appearance (eg, anterior tibiofibular ligament).

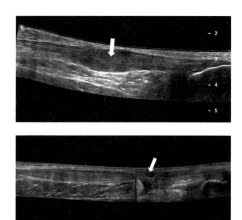

A.

B.

Figure 1-6 A, US showing severe Achilles tendinosis at its relative hypovascular (critical) zone (arrow). B, US showing acute rupture of the Achilles tendon at the critical zone (arrow).

- On US, normal ligaments have a fibrillary pattern not unlike tendons.

Ligament Tears (Sprains)

- Acutely torn ligaments are diffusely thickened with diffuse ↑SI on MRI, ±fiber discontinuity if full-thickness tear **(Fig. 1-7A)**. On US, acutely torn ligaments are diffusely thickened, heterogeneous, ±fiber discontinuity **(Fig. 1-7B)**, with surrounding edema and hyperemia on power Doppler.
- In the chronic phase, torn ligaments can have a variable appearance: Completely absent, thin/attenuated, scarred and thickened, or may appear relatively normal.

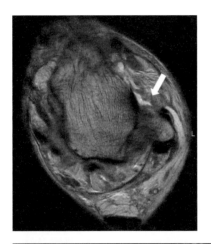

A.

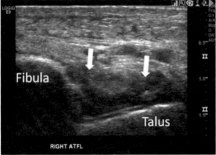

B.

Figure 1-7 Axial PD MRI (A) and US (B) showing acute complete tear of the ATFL in two different patients (arrow).

Articular Cartilage

- On MRI, hyaline cartilage is intermediate SI in most pulse sequences. PD distinguishes the different layers of hyaline cartilage as various shades of gray, most sensitive for early disorganization of collagen matrix before loss of chondral thickness.
- MRI can directly identify various stages of chondromalacia (ie, fibrillation, fissuring, chondral thinning).
- Articular cartilage layer can also be seen on US, but US not sensitive for identifying cartilage lesions.
- CT with intra-articular contrast (**arthrogram**) will outline the layer of articular cartilage and provide crude evaluation for cartilage lesions.
- X-rays cannot visualize articular cartilage, but degree of arthritis can be inferred by loss of joint space.

Osteoarthritis

- Cartilage wear accompanied by marginal osteophytes, subchondral sclerosis, and subchondral cysts, all of which could be visualized on MRI. Subchondral bone marrow edema on STIR or fat-saturated T2/PD often correlates with pain.
- Joint space narrowing, osteophytes, subchondral sclerosis, and subchondral cysts can also be seen on X-ray **(Fig. 1-8)** or CT. Some joint bodies may be more conspicuous on CT than on MRI.

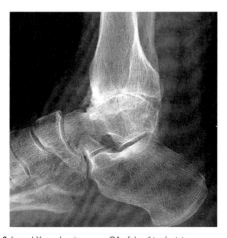

Figure 1-8 Lateral X-ray showing severe OA of the tibiotalar joint.

- US can identify osteophytes, and pressure with the transducer (sonopalpation) can assess whether the particular joint contributes to pain.
- US-guided cortisone injection into any arthritic joint will provide therapeutic relief.

Osteochondral Lesions (Osteochondritis Dissecans)

- Discrete lesions of the articular surface involving a combination of articular cartilage and subchondral bone, commonly occurring in the talar dome.
- X-ray may show a subtle lucent lesion of the subchondral bone, focal subchondral collapse, cysts, or displaced bone fragment.
- CT provides best anatomic detail of osseous involvement.
- MRI assesses both the bone and the articular cartilage **(Fig. 1-9)**; best modality for predicting instability (identifying marrow edema, cystic change and fluid at the interface, necrosis of the bone) (*Radiology* 2008;248:571).

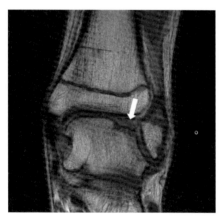

Figure 1-9 Coronal PD MRI sequence showing osteochondritis dissecans of the lateral talar dome (arrow).

SYNOVITIS/INFLAMMATORY ARTHRITIS/CRYSTAL DEPOSITION DISEASE

Synovitis

- Normal synovial lining of the joint should be thin on US and MRI and intermediate SI on all MRI pulse sequences.
- Synovitis is any inflammation of the joint. On US, will manifest as combination of joint effusion, ±synovial thickening,

and ± synovial hyperemia on power Doppler. On MRI, joint effusion, ±synovial thickening, and ± ↑SI of the synovium on T2/PD/STIR sequences.

- Differentiating the cause of synovitis on imaging is often challenging; various inflammatory arthritides (rheumatoid, sero-negative, crystal-deposition-related, septic) will present with a synovitis, and degenerative osteoarthritis (OA) can result in a reactive synovitis.
- If there is just a joint effusion in a joint with advanced OA, most likely a reactive synovitis.
- Bulky synovial hypertrophy on US/MRI with ↑SI of the synovium on T2/PD/STIR **(Fig. 1-10)** without radiographic features of OA suggests one of the inflammatory arthritides. Erosions also suggest inflammatory arthritis, although erosions can sometimes be difficult to differentiate from subchondral cysts associated with OA.

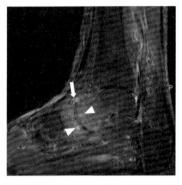

Figure 1-10 Sagittal IR MRI sequence showing talonavicular joint arthrosis with bright synovium (arrow) and erosions (arrowheads) suggestive of an inflammatory arthritis such as rheumatoid.

- Calcifications in the joint are very specific for crystal deposition disease (gout, pseudogout). X-ray and CT are sensitive for detecting calcifications. On US, bright echoes in synovium reflect microcalcifications c/w gout or pseudogout. On X-ray, chronic erosion with proliferative change of its margin (overhanging edge) with relative preservation of the joint space is hallmark of gout **(Fig. 1-11)**.

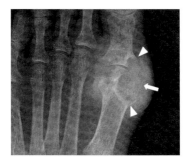

Figure I-11 Frontal radiograph of the foot demonstrates soft tissue calcification (arrow) with adjacent "overhanging edge" (arrowheads), consistent with gout.

SOFT TISSUE MASSES

- Both MRI and US provide useful and usually sufficient diagnostic information for most soft tissue masses in the foot and ankle. US has the advantage of being quick and more tolerated by the patient. On MRI, IV contrast (Gadolinium) can be given to distinguish solid from cystic lesions.

Ganglion Cyst

- Slowly growing benign fluid-filled mass due to previous micro-trauma, arising from the joint capsule, ligaments, or tendons.
- On MRI, mass that is of the same SI as fluid in all pulse sequences. Contrast usually not necessary but if given, only the lesion's peripheral pseudocapsule should enhance.
- Features typical of all cysts are seen on US: Anechoic lesion with thin imperceptible wall and increased through transmission **(Fig. I-12)**. Aspiration and rupture can be performed safely under US guidance in experienced hands, although ganglion cysts have a propensity to recur.

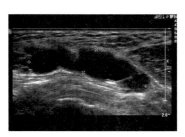

Figure I-12 US showing ganglion cyst in the tarsal tunnel located superficial to the FHL tendon.

Morton Neuroma

- Scar that forms around the plantar digital nerve at the level of the metatarsal heads, most common in the 3rd and 2nd web spaces, ±intermetatarsal bursitis.
- On MRI, teardrop-shaped mass in the characteristic location, ↓SI in all pulse sequences **(Fig. 1-13)**. Contrast is not necessary for diagnosis but will diffusely enhance if given.
- On US, hypoechoic or mixed-echogenicity mass in the web space, visible from both the plantar and dorsal aspects, which is noncompressible with gentle pressure.
- Amenable to US-guided cortisone injection.

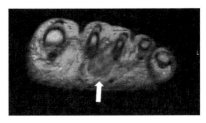

Figure 1-13 Axial PD MRI showing a Morton neuroma (arrow) of the 2nd web space.

Pigmented Villonodular Synovitis

- Benign tumor of synovium that can present in two forms: Localized and diffuse **(Fig. 1-14)**.
- ↓SI in all pulse sequences and "blooming" on gradient echo sequences on MRI are hallmark, because of hemosiderin associated with these lesions.

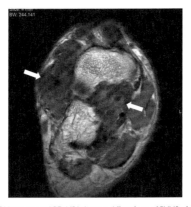

Figure 1-14 Oblique coronal PD MRI showing diffuse form of PVNS of the midfoot (arrows).

- Histologically identical lesion can involve the tendon sheath rather than the joint, called "**giant cell tumor of the tendon sheath**," which has the same MRI features other than that it involves the tendon sheath.
- On US, pigmented villonodular synovitis presents as focal mass-like area or diffuse synovial thickening, although more difficult to identify than on MRI. Giant cell tumor of the tendon sheath presents as thickened area of the tendon sheath with internal vascularity.
- If large enough, may be able to see the soft tissue prominence on CT; if the lesion contains calcifications, must consider other diagnoses.

Peripheral Nerve Sheath Tumor
- Tumor of neural elements, most are benign (**schwannoma, neurofibroma**), although small minority are malignant ("**malignant peripheral nerve sheath tumor**," typically associated with neurofibromatosis type I).
- Although the mass itself is nonspecific in appearance on MRI and US, its location within and enlarging a peripheral nerve clinches the diagnosis **(Fig. 1-15)**. MRI and US cannot provide a histologic diagnosis or assess whether the lesion is benign or malignant.

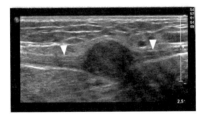

Figure 1-15 US long axis to the tibial nerve (arrowheads) in the tarsal tunnel shows mass enlarging the nerve reflecting a PNST.

Sarcomas
- Soft tissue sarcomas of the foot and ankle are exceedingly rare, and imaging cannot reliably distinguish soft tissue sarcomas from benign tumors. If a patient presents with a soft tissue mass and MRI/US does not indicate a clearly benign entity (eg, ganglion cyst), surgical excision is recommended.

BONE TUMORS

- Tumors of bone in the foot and ankle are rare and most are benign.

Unicameral Bone Cyst/Intraosseous Lipoma
- Both can rarely involve the foot, specifically the calcaneus.
- On X-ray, both manifest as a lytic lesion of the calcaneus with thin sclerotic borders without cortical destruction. A central dystrophic calcification, if present, favors lipoma over unicameral bone cyst (UBC).
- MRI will clearly distinguish between these two entities; UBC has SI of fluid **(Fig. 1-16)**, whereas lipoma has SI of fat on all pulse sequences.

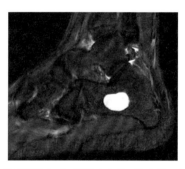

Figure 1-16 Sagittal IR MRI showing UBC in typical location in the calcaneus.

Osteoid Osteoma
- Benign tumor of bone affecting adolescents and young adults, classically causing nocturnal pain relieved with aspirin.
- Mostly involve the femur and tibia but can rarely involve small bones of the foot.
- CT is definitive imaging modality, identifying the lytic nidus in the cortex ± central calcification with a broad area of reactive cortical thickening.
- MRI shows prominent bone marrow edema and cortical thickening but the nidus itself representing the osteoid osteoma may be very subtle.
- Bone scan will show a focal lesion of ↑uptake on the skeletal phase.
- Amenable to CT-guided ablation **(Fig. 1-17)**.

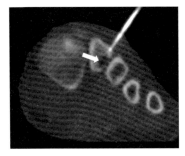

Figure 1-17 Image during CT-guided ablation shows needle being advanced toward an osteoid osteoma of the 2nd metatarsal (arrow).

INFECTION OF THE FOOT AND ANKLE

Cellulitis
- Infection of the skin and subcutaneous fat, largely a clinical diagnosis.
- MRI and US will show diffuse soft tissue edema, can R/O abscesses and bone/joint involvement. MRI will require contrast to identify soft tissue abscesses.

Soft Tissue Abscess
- Loculated fluid collection in the soft tissues, which may require incision and drainage.
- US will show a fluctuant complex fluid collection with surrounding hyperemia on power Doppler **(Fig. 1-18)**.

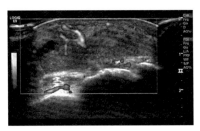

Figure 1-18 US of the dorsum of the midfoot showing a complex fluid collection with internal echoes and surrounding hyperemia on power Doppler, consistent with an abscess.

- MRI will show area of soft tissue edema ($\uparrow$SI on STIR/fat-saturated T2 or PD), but IV contrast required to identify abscess as a peripherally enhancing fluid collection.
- Sinus tracts, which are a common mode of spread of infection in diabetic feet, are also detectable on MRI only with IV contrast.

Osteomyelitis

- Bacterial seeding of bone through hematogenous spread (children, those with bacteremia) or contiguous spread (skin ulcer in diabetics). Diagnosis is important clinically because it would require long-term IV antibiotics.
- Changes not detectable on X-ray/CT for weeks. US has no role in assessing bone for osteomyelitis.
- Three-phase bone scan has high sensitivity and specificity in the appropriate clinical setting.
- On MRI, ↑SI on STIR or fat-saturated T2/PD **(Fig. 1-19)** & ↓SI on T1 is suspicious for osteomyelitis, albeit not always specific. IV contrast is not helpful in distinguishing osteomyelitis from other causes of marrow edema.

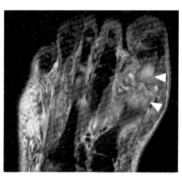

Figure 1-19 Coronal IR MRI shows septic arthritis and osteomyelitis of the 1st MTP joint (arrowheads).

Septic Arthritis

- Bacterial seeding of the joint.
- On US and MRI **(Fig. 1-19)**, imaging features can be identical to any other source of an inflammatory arthritis, although disproportionate extracapsular soft tissue edema on MRI may be more suggestive of septic arthritis. Reactive subchondral marrow edema is commonly seen across both sides of the joint, which may be indistinguishable from osteomyelitis.
- Definitive diagnosis and identification of organism will require arthrocentesis, which can be safely done under US guidance.

Septic Tenosynovitis

- Bacterial infection along a tendon within the tendon sheath, because of contiguous spread from adjacent sites of infection or from penetrating injury.
- Important to diagnose because it can lead to bacterial seeding at distant sites along the course of the involved tendon.

- On US and MRI, may be indistinguishable from tenosynovitis associated with inflammatory arthritis (eg, rheumatoid), but disproportionate subjacent soft tissue edema on MRI may suggest a septic cause.

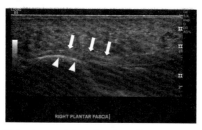

Figure 1-20 US showing normal plantar fascia (arrows) in long axis inserting on the calcaneus (arrowheads).

PLANTAR FASCIA

Normal Plantar Fascia
- Aponeurosis that arises from the plantar aspect of the calcaneus and reinforces the longitudinal arch.
- On MRI and US, thin band of tissue extending from the calcaneus to the forefoot, <3 to 4 mm thickness at the calcaneal origin **(Fig. 1-20)** (*Radiology* 1996;201:257), and homogeneously ↓SI on all MRI pulse sequences.

Plantar Fasciitis
- Thickening (>4 mm) of the plantar fascial origin at the calcaneus, with heterogeneous echotexture on US and heterogeneous ↑SI on MRI. Often with soft tissue edema in the plantar fat pad on US and MRI, ±reactive marrow edema in the calcaneus. Plantar calcaneal spur is often present.

Plantar Fascial Tear
- Partial thickness tears characteristically occur right at the calcaneal origin of the fascia in the setting of plantar fasciitis, whereas acute ruptures can occur slightly away from the calcaneal origin.
- On MRI, a linear fluid-signal cleft of the plantar fascial origin in the background of diffuse ↑SI and fascial thickening reflects a partial thickness tear. Rupture is seen as a full-thickness discontinuity with associated fusiform thickening and surrounding soft tissue edema.
- Linear hypoechoic cleft of partial thickness tear can also be appreciated on US, whereas rupture manifests as diffuse thickening, edema, and poor visualization of fascial fibers with accompanying history of recent injury **(Fig. 1-21)**.

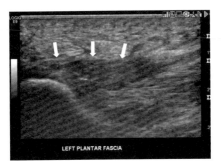

Figure 1-21 US showing acute rupture of the plantar fascia (arrows) at the calcaneal insertion in a patient who felt an acute pop in the bottom of the foot.

Plantar Fibroma

- Nodular hypertrophy of the plantar fascia that presents as a painless lump in the sole of the foot, also known as **plantar fibromatosis** and **Ledderhose disease**, and can coexist with Dupuytren contracture of the palms of the hands.
- On US, nodular thickening of the plantar fascia, often multiple, is diagnostic.
- On MRI, the masses are of heterogeneous ↑SI and can be infiltrative in appearance, although origin within the plantar fascia is highly characteristic.

PLANTAR PLATE AND SESAMOID PAIN

Normal Plantar Plate and Sesamoids

- The plantar plate is a capsuloligamentous structure that stabilizes the plantar aspects of the metatarsophalangeal joints.
- In the great toe, the hallux sesamoids and additional muscles and ligaments associated with the sesamoids result in more complex anatomy relative to the plantar plates of the lesser toes.
- On MRI, normal hallux sesamoids should have the same SI as marrow fat in all pulse sequences, and all the ligaments that reinforce the plantar plate (sesamoid-phalangeal, metatarsosesamoid, intersesamoid, and collateral ligaments) should be homogeneous ↓SI on all pulse sequences.

Turf Toe

- Hyperextension injury to the great toe, ↑prevalence among American football players after the widespread use of artificial turf.

- MRI can identify the degree of injury to the plantar plate capsuloligamentous complex, ranging from mild sprain of the plantar plate ($\uparrow$SI to the plantar plate on T2 and PD) to rupture (full-thickness defect) **(Fig. 1-22)** and retraction of the plantar plate and sesamoid-phalangeal ligaments, $\pm$chondral shear injury to the first metatarsal head.
- CT can identify osteochondral fragments or loose bodies.
- US can identify full-thickness disruption of the sesamoid-phalangeal ligaments but is not sensitive for sprains or partial thickness tears.

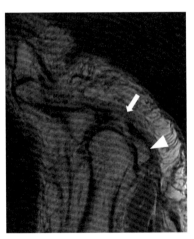

Figure 1-22 Sagittal PD MRI shows full-thickness rupture of the plantar plate (arrow) with proximal retraction of the medial sesamoid (arrowhead).

Sesamoid Pain

- **Sesamoid fracture:** Fracture line is visible on CT or MRI **(Fig. 1-23)**. MRI has the added benefit of identifying bone marrow edema ($\uparrow$SI on STIR, fat-saturated T2/PD). Fracture may sometimes be difficult to distinguish from a bipartite patella.
- **Sesamoid osteonecrosis:** Devitalized bone is diffusely $\downarrow$SI in all MRI pulse sequences **(Fig. 1-23)**, $\pm$collapse. On X-ray and CT, necrotic sesamoid is sclerotic. US has no role in assessing for osteonecrosis.
- **Sesamoiditis:** Nonspecific inflammation of the sesamoid. MRI may show marrow edema in the sesamoid without a discrete fracture line. US may show hyperemia on power Doppler, although neither sensitive nor specific.

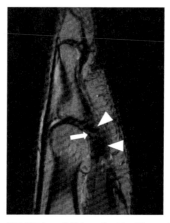

Figure 1-23 Sagittal PD MRI shows AVN (arrowheads) and fracture (arrow) of the sesamoid.

ACCESSORY BONES

- Various accessory bones can exist in the foot and ankle as a normal variant. Usually should have normal marrow SI and most are incidental findings.

Os Trigonum
- When the lateral tubercle of the posterior process of the talus remains separate from the remainder of the posterior process.
- Can be a source of posterior ankle impingement, especially in those with repetitive plantarflexion of the ankle (eg, ballet dancers).
- On MRI, bone marrow edema in the os trigonum suggests that it could be symptomatic **(Fig. 1-24)**. Fluid in the posterior recess of the ankle joint and FHL tenosynovitis can be signs of posterior ankle impingement on MRI or US. Guided injection of anesthetic ± cortisone under US around the os can confirm that it is the source of the patient's symptoms.

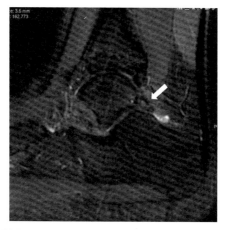

Figure 1-24 Sagittal IR MRI showing an os trigonum with a stress reaction (arrow).

Os Peroneum

- Sesamoid intimately associated with the peroneus longus tendon, can be a source of pain ("painful os peroneum syndrome"/"POPS").
- On MRI, marrow edema in the os may be seen with POPS.
- Proximal migration of the os on serial X-rays indicates rupture of the peroneus longus **(Fig. 1-25)**.
- US-guided injection into the cuboid tunnel may provide diagnostic information.

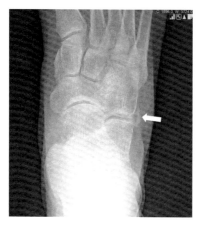

Figure 1-25 X-ray showing a fractured and proximally migrated os peroneum (arrow). Concurrent MRI showed rupture of the peroneus longus tendon (data not shown).

Accessory Navicular

- Three types (type III is a prominent cornuate process of the navicular without a separate os), located at the posterior tibialis tendon insertion. Also known as os tibiale externum.
- Can be a source of medial foot pain.
- On MRI, marrow edema within the accessory navicular and adjacent navicular is reflective of a stress reaction. Degree of posterior tibialis tendinosis can be assessed on both MRI and US.

TARSAL TUNNEL SYNDROME AND OTHER NEUROPATHIES

Tarsal Tunnel Syndrome

- Compressive neuropathy of the tibial nerve as it courses in a fibro-osseous tunnel called the tarsal tunnel.
- Imaging useful to rule out a structural source of tibial nerve compression.
- Both US and MRI can identify accessory muscles or soft tissue masses (eg, ganglion cyst) within the tarsal tunnel (**Fig. 1-26**). In the postoperative setting, US and MRI can identify neuromas of the tibial nerve and relationship of any scars with the nerve.
- Muscle denervation (muscle edema in the acute to subacute phase and fatty atrophy in the chronic phase) of the intrinsic muscles of the midfoot/forefoot is occasionally seen on MRI.
- US and MRI can also assess the two terminal branches of the tibial nerve (medial and lateral plantar nerves).

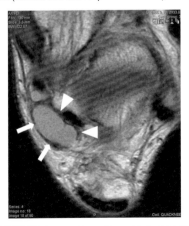

Figure 1-26 Axial PD MRI shows ganglion cyst (arrows) in the tarsal tunnel. The medial and lateral plantar nerves being compressed by the cyst are marked by arrowheads.

Other Neuropathies

- **Baxter nerve** (inferior calcaneal branch of the lateral plantar nerve) is not consistently visible on US and MRI unless there is a neuroma. There is usually no imaging correlate for **Baxter neuropathy**, which is an entrapment neuropathy. Fatty atrophy of the abductor digiti minimi muscle, historically believed to be a sign of Baxter neuropathy, is not a reliable sign because it can be present in asymptomatic individuals (*Radiology* 2009;253:160).
- **Joplin neuroma**, an entrapment neuropathy of the medial plantar proper digital nerve to the hallux, usually does not have an imaging correlate, although the nerve itself can be seen both on US and MRI.
- **Superficial peroneal nerve entrapment** is believed to occur because it pierces the deep fascia in the distal third of the leg. Although there is usually not an imaging correlate unless there is a neuroma **(Fig. I-27)**, the nerve itself can be clearly visualized on US and MRI and US can be used to guide diagnostic injections.
- US-guided injection of anesthetic ± cortisone may provide diagnostic information for patients presenting with tarsal tunnel syndrome or other neuropathies.

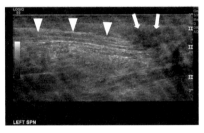

Figure I-27 US of the distal calf/ankle shows stump neuroma (arrows) of the superficial peroneal nerve (arrowheads).

TARSAL COALITION

- Congenital fusion of two tarsal bones, occurring as three types (osseous, cartilaginous, fibrous). Any joint of the foot/ankle can be involved, but vast majority are either talocalcaneal or calcaneonavicular.
- On X-ray, pes planus with secondary signs, such as the "C-sign" and "talar beak," can suggest talocalcaneal coalition.
- Bone scans will show increased tracer uptake at sites of symptomatic coalition.

- CT provides better anatomic detail and can distinguish between osseous and non-osseous types of coalition **(Fig. 1-28)**.
- MRI will also distinguish between osseous and non-osseous; presence of marrow edema (↑SI on STIR, fat-saturated T2/PD) suggests a stress reaction, and osseous irregularity at the coalition site suggests a pseudoarthrosis.

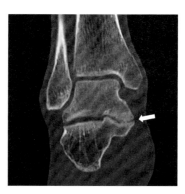

Figure 1-28 Coronal reformation of a CT scan shows non-osseous talocalcaneal tarsal coalition (arrow).

PHYSICAL EXAMINATION

SCOTT YATES

OVERVIEW

When examining the foot, consider the multiple systems represented in it. The exam will focus on four systems. **Even if complaint is unilateral, always examine both feet.**

Basic Foot Exam			
Vascular	**Neurologic**	**Dermatologic**	**Musculoskeletal**
Pulses	Vibratory sensation	Skin color/ texture/turgor	Sitting/standing
Capillary refill	Position sense	Scaling	Neutral/pes planus/pes cavus
Elevation/ dependency	Light touch	Interspaces	Muscle strength
Swelling	Protective sensation	Hydrated/dry/ fissures	ROM
Temperature gradient	Reflexes	Corns/callus/ fat pad	Gait exam
Venous filling time	Plantar response	Nail plates	Shoe exam

VASCULAR EXAM

- **Visual inspection**/skin changes/varicosities/pigmentation/ quality of skin
- **Pulses** (femoral/popliteal/posterior tibial/dorsalis pedis)
  - **Femoral:** Mid-inguinal point below inguinal ligament
  - **Popliteal:** with knee flexed, place hands on front of knee and palpate in popliteal space
  - **Posterior tibial:** Posterior to medial malleolus
  - **Dorsalis pedis:** Dorsum of foot lateral to EHL
  Grading system (with 4 as denominator)

0/4	1/4	2/4	3/4	4/4
Absent	Diminished	Weak but palpable	Easily palpable	Bounding

  If not palpable, can use handheld Doppler
- **Capillary refill**
  Normal is **less than or equal to 2 seconds.** Prolonged capillary refill may be an indicator of peripheral arterial disease (PAD).
- **Elevation/dependency**
  Check for **pallor on elevation/rubor on dependency**

- **Swelling**
  Grade swelling on scale of +1 to +4. Is it **pitting or nonpitting?**
- **Temperature gradient**
  Gradient measured with back of hand from anterior aspect of leg (shin) to dorsum of foot
  - **Normal:** Foot cooler than leg by about 6°
  - **Increased:** Foot cooler than anterior aspect of leg by >6°. May be sign of PAD.
  - **Reversed:** Foot warmer than anterior aspect of leg. May be sign of inflammation or infection.
- **Venous filling time**
  Test for arterial insufficiency. Mark vein on dorsum of foot. Elevate extremity for 1 minute or until vein has drained. Place limb in dependent position. Record time it takes for vein to refill. **Normal is less than 20 seconds.**

  If vascular examination suggests possibility of PAD, consider referral to vascular lab for **L**ower **E**xtremity **N**oninvasive testing (**LENI**s). Test may include arterial Doppler, PVR, segmental plethysmography, ABI, TCPO$_2$.

NEUROLOGIC EXAM

- **Vibratory sensation:** Place tuning fork on medial 1st metatarsal head or malleolus. Ask patient to "tell me when you stop feeling it vibrate." Patient should perceive vibration to stop as about same time as you feel vibration stop.
- **Position sense:** Done with patient's eyes closed. Grasp hallux from side. Dorsiflex/plantar flex toe. Ask patient if toe is "going up or going down."
- **Sharp/dull**
- **Light touch:** With wisp of cotton
- **10 g monofilament wire:** Test for protective sensation
- **Reflexes:** Achilles/patella

0	1+	2+	3+	4+	5+
Absent	Trace	Normal	Brisk	Nonsustained clonus	Sustained clonus

- **Plantar response**
  - **Normal**—toes going down
  - **Absent**
  - **Abnormal/Babinski**—great toe goes up/fanning of lesser toes. **There is no such thing as a "negative Babinski."**

DERMATOLOGIC EXAM

- **Skin color:** Check for areas of increased/decreased pigmentation
- **Skin texture:** Normal or atrophic and shiny
- **Skin turgor:** Assess elasticity of skin
- **Scaling:** Look for patterns of scaling (moccasin distribution-tinea pedis)
- **Interspaces:** Dry or macerated
- **Hydration:** Is skin appropriately moisturized?
- **Fat pad:** Anterior displacement or fat pad atrophy
- **Corns and calluses:** Presence or absence/location
- **Fissures:** Check heels and interdigital spaces
- **Nail plates:** Are nail plates dystrophic, attached to nail bed, evidence of subungual debris, pitting, subungual bleeding, color

---

MUSCULOSKELETAL EXAM

- **Examine feet** with patient both **sitting and standing** (weight bearing/off weight bearing)
- **Foot type:** Neutral, pes planus, pes cavus
- **Pes planus:** Flexible or rigid. "Too many toes" sign. Seen with pronation when foot viewed from behind, appears to have extra toes
- **Cavus foot** (high arch): The etiology of a cavus foot may be idiopathic, but may often be associated with underlying neurologic disease (think CMT, post CVA, post-polio). Unilateral cavus foot should always increase concern for neurologic etiology.
- **Types of cavus feet**
  - **Rigid:** No change in shape from sitting to standing
  - **Semi-rigid:** Flattens when standing, but maintains shape of arch
  - **Flexible:** High arched when sitting, no arch when standing; functions as flatfoot
- **Muscle strength**
  - Dorsiflexion (tibialis anterior)
  - Plantar flexion (gastrocnemius)
  - Inversion/plantar flexion (posterior tibial)
  - Eversion/dorsiflexion (peroneals)
- **Grading scale (Oxford scale)**
  - 0/5 No contraction
  - 1/5 Visible/palpable muscle contraction, but no movement
  - 2/5 Movement with gravity eliminated
  - 3/5 Movement against gravity only

- 4/5 Movement against gravity with some resistance
- 5/5 Movement against gravity with full resistance
- **ROM**
  - **Ankle joint:** dorsiflexion/plantar flexion, 0° to 20° dorsiflexion/0° to 15° plantar flexion
  - **Subtalar joint/midtarsal joint:** 2/3 inversion/1/3 eversion
  - **MTP joints:** Dorsiflexion/plantar flexion
  - **IP joints:** Dorsiflexion/plantar flexion
  - Is there full ROM or limited ROM? Is there evidence of crepitus? Is there pain on ROM?
- **Gastrocsoleus equinus (Silverskiold test)**
  Test with knee extended/knee flexed. 10° ankle dorsiflexion with knee extended/if no, does it increase with knee flexed?
- **Gait examination**
  If presenting complaint is musculoskeletal, may want to perform a more detailed gait exam. If not a musculoskeletal complaint, perform a basic gait evaluation. This can be done in the treatment room, if space permits, or in an adjacent hallway. Start by looking at the head and then progressively scan down to feet. As the patient is walking, evaluate shoulder position, arm swing, hip position, and knee position. Look at foot position at heel strike, midstance, and toe off. Look for any asymmetry in gait. Can also watch gait as patient walks in/out of treatment room.
- **Shoe exam**
  Look for wear patterns on sole of shoe. Shoe should be wide enough and long enough to fit the foot. Draw outline of patient's foot (without shoe on) on piece of paper. Draw outline of shoe on another piece of paper. Does outline of foot "fit" comfortably into outline of shoe? If not, visual evidence of foot-shoe incompatibility. Shoe may be contributing factor to foot complaint.

PROBLEM-FOCUSED EXAM

- **Verruca**
  - Pinpoint capillary bleeding
  - Interruption of skin lines
  - Pain with compression and direct palpation
- **Callus**
  - No capillary bleeding
  - No interruption of skin lines
  - Pain with direct palpation only

- **Neuroma**
  - Palpate at level of affected interspace
  - Compression of forefoot and palpation at interspace
  - **Palpable/audible click:** Mulder sign
- **Plantar fasciitis versus heel fracture**
  In fracture, squeezing calcaneus elicits pain
- **Metatarsal stress fracture**
  Tuning fork over presumed fracture site elicits pain

SUGGESTED READINGS

Alazzawi S, Sukeik M, King D, Vemulapalli K. Foot and ankle history and clinical examination: a guide to everyday practice. *World J Orthop.* 2017;8(1):21-29.

DeOrio JK, Shapiro SA, McNeil RB. Validity of posterior tibial edema sign in posterior tibial tendon dysfunction. *Foot Ankle Int.* 2011;32(2):189-192.

SATWINDER KAUR GOSAL

PRINCIPLES OF PHYSICAL THERAPY

- **Strengthening exercises**
  - **Isometric:** Contraction against a fixed resistance, no motion
  - **Isotonic:** Weight moved through a range of motion, dynamic contraction
    - **Concentric:** Shortening. Positive work
    - **Eccentric:** Lengthening. Negative work
  - **Isokinetic:** Time-controlled resistance. Contraction at constant velocity with use of bar or device with adjustable resistance
- **Cryotherapy:** Use of cold in the tx and rehab of MSK injuries and conditions
  - **Methods:** Cold packs, ice massage, cold spray, immersion, cold compression units, cryokinetics
  - **Physiologic effects:** Vasoconstriction, ↓cellular metabolism, ↓swelling, analgesia, ↓muscle spasm/spasticity, reduced muscle spindle excitability, reactive hyperemia, Hunting Rxn
  - **Indications:** Muscle spasm, trauma, inflammation, swelling, pain
  - **Contraindications:** Impaired sensory perception, cold allergy, Raynaud, vascular disease, h/o pernio or frostbite, RA, cryoglobulinemia
- **Thermotherapy**
  - Different forms
    - **Superficial:** <1 cm depth penetration.
      - Hot air, paraffin, infrared, whirlpool, hot packs, radiant light, hot water
    - **Deep:** 2 to 5 cm depth penetration
      - Short wave diathermy, ultrasound, microwave diathermy
  - **Physiologic effects:** Vasodilation, ↑capillary permeability, ↑local tissue metabolism, ↓joint stiffness, ↑circulation, analgesia, hyperemia, ↑tissue temp, ↓muscle spasm
  - **Indications:** Arthritis, stiff joints, muscle spasms, trauma, pain, inflammation
  - **Contraindications:** Acute trauma, PVD, heat sensitivity/insensitivity, malignancies, febrile conditions, malignancy, pregnancy (deep tx), pacemaker (deep tx)

- **Electrical stimulation**
  - **Iontophoresis:** Noninvasive delivery of chemicals (anesthetic or anti-inflammatory) of like charge through skin. Direct current
  - **Phonophoresis:** Noninvasive delivery of chemicals through ultrasound

BIOMECHANICS (ORTHOTICS, BRACING, AND PADDING)

- **Orthotic:** In-shoe device utilized to assist, resist, stabilize, or improve ROM and functional capacity
  - **Functional foot orthosis:** Orthotic custom or prefab that treats mechanical pathologies of the foot
  - **Accommodative foot orthosis:** Orthotic custom or prefab to offload and accommodate areas of pressure and deformity
- **Posting:** Increase support of heel of an orthotic, stabilize foot against ground reactive forces, tilt contoured plate against foot
- **Dancer's pad:** Used to off-weight 1st met head: sesamoiditis or fx'd sesamoid
- **Heel lift:** tx apophysitis, LLD, equinus, plantar fasciitis, Haglund deformity
- **Morton extension:** Limit 1st MTPJ ROM, hallux limitus, hallux rigidus
- **Reverse Morton extension:** Increase 1st ray ROM
- **Metatarsal bar/pad:** Placed behind met heads to transfer pressure off met head 2, 3, and 4
- **Low dye strap:** Strapping technique achieved with tape to reduce strain associated with pronation
- **Bracing**
  - **AFOs:** Ankle set at 90°. Tx: drop foot, ankle arthritis, equinus, NM disease causes equinus
  - **CROW:** Charcot Restraint Orthotic Walker

EXTRACORPOREAL SHOCKWAVE THERAPY

- **Technology:** High-energy sound waves to treat MSK conditions
- **Indications:** Soft tissue injuries, plantar fasciitis, Achilles tendonitis, acute and chronic muscle pain
- **Contraindication:** DVT, malignancy, pacemakers, cortisone injections within 1 month prior to the start of therapy, pregnancy

BIOLOGICS

- **Platelet-rich plasma therapy:** Injection therapy consisting of autologous platelets
- **Mesenchymal stem cell therapy:** MSC extracted from bone marrow aspirate, used in conjunction with PRP

SUGGESTED READINGS

Kannus P, Renstrom P. Treatment for acute tears of the lateral ligaments of the ankle. Operation, cast, or early controlled mobilization. *J Bone Joint Surg Am.* 1991;73:305-312.

Pfeffer G, Bacchetti P, Deland J, et al. Comparison of custom and prefabricated orthoses in the initial treatment of proximal plantar fasciitis. *Foot Ankle Int.* 1999;20(4):214-221.

PERIOPERATIVE CONSIDERATIONS

JARED WORTZMAN

RISK ASSESSMENT/OPTIMIZATION

- **ASA physical status classification:** Not meant as risk assessment tool to predict outcomes, but rather general classification of patient physical status. The edition of "E" to classification status denotes emergency surgery.

ASA Physical Status Classification		
ASA Class	**Definition**	**Examples**
ASA I	Disease-free patient	Healthy, nonsmoker
ASA II	Mild systemic disease	Smoker, controlled HTN or DM, obesity
ASA III	Severe systemic disease with functional limitations	Poorly controlled HTN or DM, ESRD with regular dialysis, stable history of CAD
ASA IV	Severe systemic disease that is a constant threat to life	Recent MI, CVA, CAD/stents (<3 mo), severe valvular disease, ESRD not on dialysis
ASA V	Patient not expected to survive without surgery	Massive trauma, ruptured aortic aneurysm, intracranial bleed with mass effect
ASA VI	Brain dead patient; surgery for organ donation	

- **Basic preoperative assessment**
  - **History:** Focus on cardiac (HTN, CAD, CHF), pulmonary (OSA, pHTN, COPD), prior experience with anesthesia; ↑perioperative risk w/↑ comorbidities. ASA Physical Status Score: Categorizes patients by baseline medical status, NOT absolute predictor of risk
  - **Exam:** Includes assessment of airway, heart (murmurs, signs of CHF), lungs, BMI, vascular access
  - **Lab/studies:** Driven by H&P/planned procedure; often includes EKG, baseline labs (hematocrit, coagulation, renal function)
- **Medications:** Most cardiac meds, insulin, inhalers should be taken day of surgery; **ASA/Plavix** warrants discussion with cardiologist (consider indication for med, eg, 1° vs 2° prevention, stents)

FASTING STATUS

- Goal to ↓ risk of pulmonary aspiration
- Risk ↑ with delayed gastric emptying from causes such as diabetes, obesity, pregnancy, GERD, opioid use

Fasting Guidelines	
Type of Food	**Recommended Fasting Time**
Clear liquids (eg, water, coffee/tea, **no milk**)	>2 h
Solid foods or non-clear liquids	>6 h
Fatty foods and meat	>8 h

Note: OK to give most medications po with small sip of water
ASA Practice Guidelines for Preoperative Fasting Anesthesiology. 1999;90:896-905; updated 2011.

ANTIBIOTIC PROPHYLAXIS

- Surgical site infections in clean procedures primarily caused by skin flora (strep and staph species)
- **Skin antiseptics:** Chlorhexidine > iodine to ↓ SSI (superficial and deep incision) *(NEJM 2010;362:18)*
- Standard of care includes antibiotic prophylaxis for all orthopedic procedures, typically with cefazolin (given within 60 min of incision).
- **Contaminated/dirty wounds:** Antibiotics should be given as treatment tailored to expected organisms, NOT as prophylaxis.

VENOUS THROMBOEMBOLISM

- **Risk factors:** Prior history, ↑age, ↑BMI, active malignancy
- ↑Risk with major orthopedic procedure, though risk less clear for minor lower limb procedures. Prophylactic anticoagulation with LMWH for less extensive lower extremity procedures is likely unnecessary *(POT-KAST/POT-CAST NEJM 2017;376(6):515)*
- **Atrial fibrillation:** In patients on Coumadin, bridging with LMWH has no change on arterial thromboembolism, ↑risk of major bleeding *(BRIDGE NEJM 2015;373(9):823):* Anticoagulation for other indications (eg, mechanical valve, prothrombotic disorders) warrants careful consideration of risk versus benefit.

SUGGESTED READINGS

Hanslow SS, Grujic L, Slater HK. Thromboembolic disease after foot and ankle surgery. *Foot Ankle Int.* 2006;27(9):693-695.

Krannitz KW, Fong HW, Fallat LM. The effect of cigarette smoking on radiographic bone healing after elective foot surgery. *J Foot Ankle Surg.* 2009;48(5):525-527.

Wukich DK, Crim BE, Frykberg RG. Neuropathy and poorly controlled diabetes increase the rate of surgical site infection after foot and ankle surgery. *J Bone Joint Surg Am.* 2014;96(10):832-839.

ANESTHESIA

JARED WORTZMAN

CHOICE OF ANESTHESIA

- Should be made in consultation with the surgeon, anesthesiologist, and patient
- **Factors to consider:** Patient comorbidities, anticipated length of case, experience of anesthesia provider, anticipated surgical pain
- Often a combination of local and regional anesthesia sufficient for foot and ankle procedures

LOCAL ANESTHESIA

- Produces effects via sodium channel blockade
- ↓pain scores, ↓opioid requirement
- **Two types:** Esters and amides (amides overwhelmingly used)
- **Risks:** Rare; primarily related to systemic toxicity at high doses or intravascular injection

Common Local Anesthetics			
Name	Onset (min)	Duration (h)	Max Dose (w/epi)
Lidocaine	2-5	2-3	5 mg/kg (7 mg/kg)
Mepivacaine	10-20	3-6	5 mg/kg (7 mg/kg)
Ropivacaine	10-30	3-15	3 mg/kg
Bupivacaine	15-30	6-8	2.5 mg/kg (3 mg/kg)

REGIONAL ANESTHESIA

- **Neuraxial anesthesia:** Spinal and epidural
  - Typically provides full anesthesia of the lower extremities; more commonly used for joint replacement
  - **Risks/complications:** Sympathetic block (↓HR, ↓BP), headache, urinary retention
  - Given high morbidity of epidural hematoma, may be contraindicated if DVT prophylaxis, anticoagulation required
- **Common peripheral nerve blocks:** Deep local anesthetic injections targeted to specific peripheral nerves
  - **Femoral:** Blocks anteromedial thigh and medial leg; limited use in isolation for below-knee procedures
  - **Saphenous:** Continuation of femoral nerve; limited use in isolation

- **Sciatic:** In combination with femoral block provides near-complete lower extremity anesthesia
- **Popliteal:** Provides coverage of the sciatic nerve territories below the knee; in combination with femoral block provides near-complete below-knee anesthesia
- **Ankle:** Anesthetic applied circumferentially at the level of the malleoli; can block entire sensory nerve supply to the foot
- **Mayo:** Anesthetic applied circumferentially along the base of the metatarsal; useful for metatarsal osteotomies
- **Digital:** Anesthetic applied both medially and laterally along the base of select digit; provides anesthesia for isolated digit
  For foot and ankle procedures not requiring tourniquet, femoral/popliteal block or ankle block often sufficient

GENERAL ANESTHESIA

- Loss of consciousness during which patient is unarousable to even painful stimuli
- Typically not necessary for elective foot and ankle procedures
- Has more significant effects on cardiovascular system, and can have lingering effects, including impaired cognition (particularly in the elderly), nausea, vomiting
- **Common agents**
  - **Propofol:** IV agent with rapid onset and elimination; provides some antiemetic effect; useful for induction of anesthesia, maintenance of anesthesia, and procedural sedation; can cause hypotension
  - **Nitrous oxide:** Inhaled gas with rapid onset and elimination; associated with significant postoperative nausea
  - **Volatiles (Isoflurane, Sevoflurane):** Inhaled agents with variable pharmacokinetics; provide amnesia, immobility; can produce cardiovascular depression and nausea

MUSCLE RELAXATION

- Requires mechanical ventilation
- Need for muscle relaxation will depend on surgeon, planned procedure
- **Depolarizing NMB drugs:** Succinylcholine; rapid onset, short duration of access; many side effects including hyperkalemia
- **Nondepolarizing NMB drugs:** curoniums; variable onset and duration; renal clearance (except cisatracurium); should be reversed
  Nondepolarizing NMB drugs typically reversed with Neostigmine, which causes bradycardia; pretreatment w/antimuscarinic is typical

POSTOPERATIVE CONSIDERATIONS

- **Postoperative nausea and vomiting**
  - **Risk factors:** Female, younger age, nonsmoker, history of PONV, history of motion sickness, inhaled anesthetics or NO; ↑incidence with ↑# of risk factors
  - **Prevention:** Multimodal approach should be employed including ↓ use of opioids; in general, can treat with one fewer agents than # risk factors

Common Antiemetic Agents		
Type of Agent	**Timing of Administration**	**Example**
Low PONV risk anesthesia	Throughout case	TIVA w/propofol regional anesthesia
Anticholinergics	Prior to induction	Scopolamine patch
Glucocorticoids	Postinduction	Dexamethasone
Serotonin antagonists	Prior to emergence	Ondansetron
Dopamine antagonists	Prior to emergence	Haloperidol

- **Pain control:** Good postoperative pain control → early mobilization, improved outcome
  Employ a multimodal approach
  - **Oral nonopioid medications:** Include acetaminophen, NSAIDs (ibuprofen), membrane stabilizers (gabapentin, pregabalin)
    All shown to decrease postoperative opioid consumption when used as adjuncts
  - **Opioid medications:** Typically given intravenously as part of induction, as well as intraoperatively
    - **Risks:** ↑PONV, respiratory depression, sedation, urinary retention, constipation; **use with caution in elderly patients**
    - **Use opioids with caution:** Patients prescribed opioids postoperatively have >5% likelihood of still using opioids at 1 year; risk ↑ w/↑ duration of therapy, long-acting medications (*MMWR* 2017;66:265). Similar rates have been observed with tramadol.
  - **Local and regional anesthesia:** Can be used pre- or postoperatively
    - **Risks:** rare; primarily related to systemic toxicity; **regional anesthesia (eg, peripheral nerve blocks) is quite user dependent**
    - **Benefits:** can allow for maintenance of consciousness; ↓opioid requirements

HALLUX ABDUCTO VALGUS

PATRICK JORDAN

HALLUX ABDUCTO VALGUS

- The most common forefoot deformity (*Orthopade* 2017;46:283)
- Deformity with lateral transverse plane deviation and abductory frontal plane deviation of the hallux
- Seen more often in women and those >65 years of age

ETIOLOGY

Exact cause has yet to be identified but believed to result from multiple factors.
- Shoe gear
- Genetics
- Ligamentous laxity
- Spastic disorders (eg, cerebral palsy)
- Inflammatory joint disorders (eg, SLE, gout)
- Abnormal 1st MPJ anatomy
- Abnormal biomechanics
- Previous foot surgery

BIOMECHANICAL EVALUATION

Static Exam
Examine:
- 1st IPJ position and ROM
- 1st MPJ position and ROM
- Tracking versus track bound
- Medial dorsal 1st metatarsal bump associated with pain, erythema
- Metatarsus adductus
- 1st ray dorsiflexion/plantarflexion
- 1st metatarsal—medial cuneiform hypermobility
- Ligamentous laxity
- Ankle ROM for equinus

Gait Exam
Evaluate:
- 1st ray position
- Arch height

- **Ankle dorsiflexion:** Is there early heel off indicating shortening of triceps surae?
- Angle and base of gait
- Antalgic gait pattern

RADIOGRAPHIC EVALUATION

- IM < 8
- Hallux abductus angle < 15
- HAI < 10
- Tibial sesamoid position 1 to 3
- Metatarsus adductus < 15
- PASA < 8
- DASA < 8
- 1st metatarsal protrusion ± 2 mm
- Osteopenia
- DJD
- Bone cysts

CONSERVATIVE TREATMENT

- Icing
- NSAIDs
- Night splints
- Accommodative shoe gear
- Orthotics
- Taping
- Stretching/manipulation

SURGICAL TREATMENT

Lateral Release
1. Release of the adductor hallucis from the lateral fibular sesamoid and lateral proximal phalanx
2. Release of the fibular metatarsal-fibular sesamoid ligament
3. Lateral flexor hallucis brevis tenotomy between the lateral sesamoid and the proximal phalanx base
4. Fibular sesamoidectomy (can lead to hallux varus) (*McGlamry* 2013;1:245)

Proximal Phalanx Procedures
- **Distal akin:** Corrects HAI
- **Proximal akin:** Corrects DASA

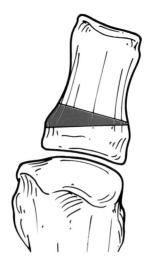

Distal 1st Metatarsal Procedures
- **Silver:** Medial "bumpectomy"
- **Modified McBride:** Soft tissue release and resection of the 1st metatarsal medial eminence
- **Austin:** Chevron osteotomy, angle of 60°

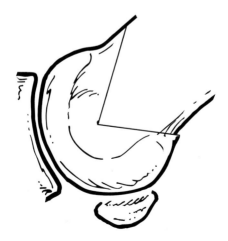

- **Youngswick:** Chevron osteotomy with removal of dorsal wedge for correction of IM and elevatus

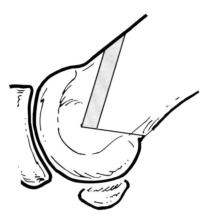

- **Reverdin:** Corrects PASA, leaves the lateral cortex intact

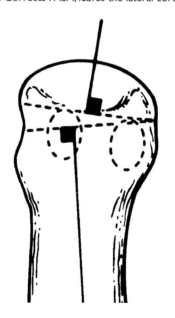

- **Reverdin-Green:** Corrects PASA, leaves the sesamoidal articulation intact by utilizing a distal "L" osteotomy

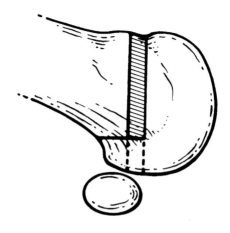

- **Reverdin-Laird:** Corrects PASA, IM. Same as Reverdin-Green, but breaks through the lateral cortex and the metatarsal head is shifted laterally

1st Metatarsal Shaft Procedures
- **Kalish:** Long-arm Austin, angle of 55°

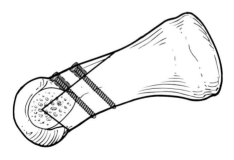

- **Scarf:** Distal and proximal cuts are made at an angle of 60° from the longitudinal cut. The metatarsal head is translated laterally 6 to 10 mm.

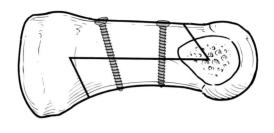

1st Metatarsal Base Procedures
- **Crescentic:** Does not shorten the metatarsal
- Closing base wedge osteotomy (CBWO)
- Opening base wedge osteotomy
- **Logroscino:** CBWO with reverdin

1st Metatarsal-Cuneiform Joint Procedures
- **Lapidus arthrodesis:** Hypermobility. Fusion of 1st metatarsal-medial cuneiform joint

Procedure indication based on IM angle		
Mild IM (8-11)	**Moderate IM (12-15)**	**Severe IM (>16)**
Silver	Austin	Crescentic
Lateral release	Reverdin-Laird/Todd	CBWO
Modified McBride	Kalish	OBWO
	Youngswick	Lapidus
	Off-set V/Vogler	
	Scarf	

Abbreviations
HAV = Hallux abducto valgus
IM = IM angle
HAI = Hallux abductus interphalangeus angle
PASA = proximal articular set angle
DASA = distal articular set angle

HALLUX LIMITUS AND HALLUX RIGIDUS

MANOJ SADHNANI • DINA IBRAHIM

Normal 1st MTPJ ROM needed for gait (Root et al., 1977) DF 65° to 75°, PF 40°
- **Hallux limitus:** Decreased ROM at the 1st MTPJ
- **Hallux rigidus:** Absence of motion at the 1st MTPJ (end stage of hallux limitus)

ETIOLOGY

- 1st Metatarsal elevatus: Acquired: hypermobile 1st ray (varus deformity–forefoot varus, rearfoot varus)
- Excessive long 1st ray
- 1st metatarsal elevatus (congenital)
- DJD:
  1. Osteoarthritis
  2. Traumatic arthritis
  3. Systemic arthritis

CLASSIFICATION

Regnauld (1986)
- **Grade I:** Functional limitation of dorsiflexion, mild dorsal spurring, pain derived from dorsal hypertrophy, no structural sesamoid disease
- **Grade II:** Broadening and flattening of metatarsal head and base of proximal phalanx, joint space narrowing, structural 1st ray elevatus, osteochondral defect, sesamoid hypertrophy
- **Grade III:** Severe loss of joint space; extensive dorsal, medial, and lateral spurring; osteochondral defects of metatarsal head and/or proximal phalanx, with or without joint mice; extensive sesamoid hypertrophy; and loss of joint space, near ankylosis

Coughlin and Shurnas (1999)
- **Grade 0:** DF of 40° to 60° (20% loss of normal motion), normal radiographic results, and no pain
- **Grade 1:** DF of 30° to 40°, dorsal osteophytes, and minimal to no other joint changes

- **Grade 2:** DF of 10° to 30°, mild flattening of the MTP joint, mild to moderate joint space narrowing or sclerosis, and osteophytes
- **Grade 3:** DF of less than 10°, often less than 10° PF, severe radiographic changes with hypertrophied cysts or erosions or with irregular sesamoids, constant moderate to severe pain, and pain at the extremes of ROM
- **Grade 4:** Stiff joint, radiographs showing loose bodies or osteochondral defects, and pain throughout entire ROM (*Foot Ankle Int* 24:661-672)

SIGNS AND SYMPTOMS

- Pain within the 1st MTPJ and dorsally over the joint
- Stiffness of the 1st MTPJ
- Dorsal prominence
- Spastic EHL
- Pinch callus at IPJ
- Paresthesia
- Gait alterations
  1. Early heel lift
  2. Apropulsive gait

RADIOGRAPHIC FINDINGS (AP, LATERAL)

- Nonuniform joint space narrowing 1st MTPJ
- Flattening of the 1st metatarsal head
- Osteophytes on 1st metatarsal head and base of proximal phalanx (aka dorsal flag sign)
- Subchondral sclerosis and subchondral cyst
- Loose bodies (joint mice) within the 1st ray
- **Elevated first metatarsal:** Lateral projection

CONSERVATIVE TREATMENT

- **Physical therapy:** Joint manipulation
- Shoe modifications
  1. **Rocker-bottom shoes:** Contribute to 1st MPJ DF limitation
  2. **Metatarsal bars:** Transfer weight over the bar at heel off to avoid DF stress on the 1st MPJ
- **Orthotics:** Posting to decrease abnormal pronation with addition of 1st ray cutout or Morton extension
- Kinetic wedge causes plantar flexion of the 1st ray
- Intra-articular corticosteroid injections
- NSAIDs

Joint Preserving Procedures
- **Soft tissue releases:** Medial band of plantar fascia, FHB, sesamoids
- Removal of the osteophytic proliferation

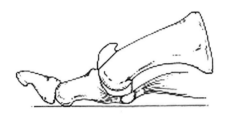

- **Watermann osteotomy:** Removal of a dorsally trapezoidal wedge osteotomy of the 1st metatarsal head and neck area to allow dorsiflexion of the hallux

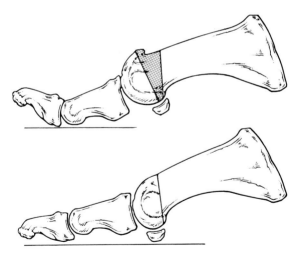

- **Modified Watermann osteotomy:** A triangular wedge of bone maintaining the integrity of plantar cortex and cartilage

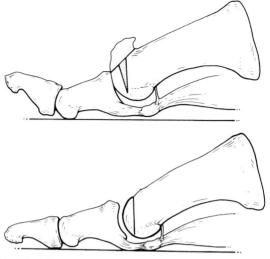

- **Modified Green:** Watermann osteotomy: removal of a rectangular section of bone. Enlarging the angle between the dorsal and plantar cuts results in further plantar flexion of the capital fragment for enhanced weight-bearing function. Two cuts:
  - **Dorsal cut:** Trapezoid wedge
  - **Plantar cut:** Oblique osteotomy

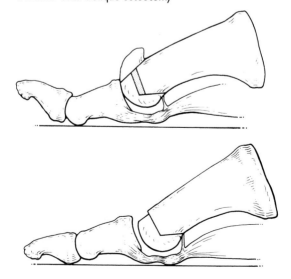

- **Youngswick-Austin procedure:** Shortens and PF the 1st metatarsal head. Two parallel cuts are made dorsally to remove a segment of bone.

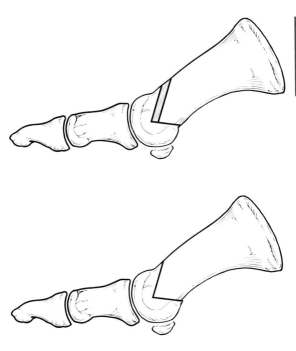

Lambrinudi osteotomy (plantarflexory wedge osteotomy): Resection of an oblique wedge of bone to correct metatarsus primus elevatus

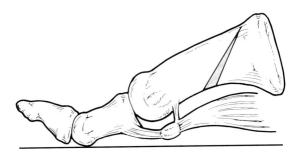

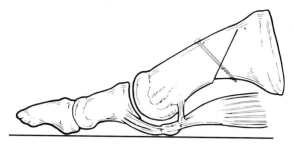

- **Kessel-Bonney osteotomy:** Involves resection of a dorsally based wedge of bone from the base of the proximal phalanx of the hallux

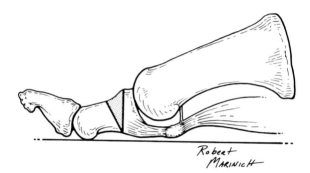

Robert
MARINICH

Joint Destructive Procedures

- **Keller arthroplasty:** Resection of one-third of the proximal phalangeal base

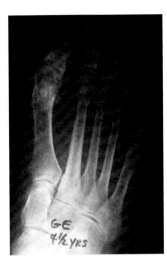

- **Mayo-Stone:** The Mayo-Stone procedure involves an angular resection of bone from the metatarsal head.
- **McKeever arthrodesis:** Fusion of the metatarsal-phalangeal joint that involves spearing the head of the metatarsal head into the base of the proximal phalanx

   Joint fixation methods involve use of lag screws, dorsal plating, bone staples, Kirschner wires, cerclage wire loops, and a combination of lag screw and dorsal plating, locking screws (ie, osteoporotic joint) (*Foot Ankle Int* 27:869-876).

  - **Frontal plane:** 0°: hallux is placed in neutral in the frontal plane.
  - **Transverse plane:** 10°: hallux should not be overly abducted permitting touching, underlapping, or overlapping of the second toe.
  - **Sagittal plane:** 10° to 15° to the floor, 20° to 25° from metatarsal: Hallux is placed in a slightly more dorsiflexed than neutral position relative to the weight-bearing surface, which encourages weight-bearing forces through the later phases of gait.

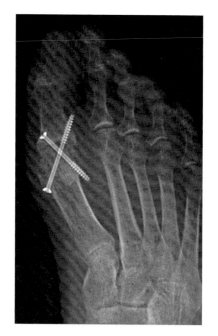

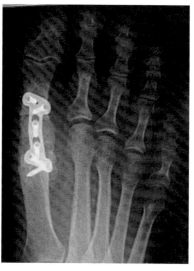

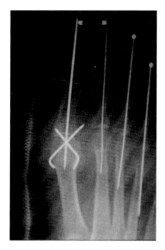

- **Valenti arthroplasty:** Involves angular resection from both the metatarsal head and the proximal phalanx
- Implant arthroplasty (total or hemi-implant)

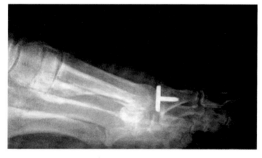

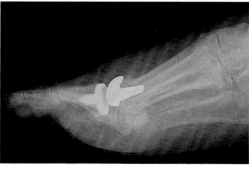

Implant Arthroplasty vs. Joint Destructive Procedures	
Indications for Implant Arthroplasty	**Joint Destructive Alternatives**
Hallux rigidus: late stage III, stage IV	Resection arthroplasty
Hallux valgus with degenerative arthritis	Interpositional implant arthroplasty
	Hemi-metallic implant
Rheumatoid arthritis	Hinged silicone implant
Revisionary first MPJ surgery with joint arthrosis or osseous deficit	Total joint replacement
	Arthrodesis
Traumatic arthritis	

From Southerland JT, Vickers DF, Boberg JS. *McGlamry's Comprehensive Textbook of Foot and Ankle Surgery.* 4th ed. Philadelphia, PA: Lippincott Williams & Wilkins; 2013.

POSTOPERATIVE MANAGEMENT

- Protected weight bearing with surgical shoes or CAM walker may be allowed after distal osteotomies and joint fusion.
- NWB at least 6 weeks after proximal osteotomies
- Physical therapy: Decreased post op adhesions
- Orthotics and accommodative devices

HAMMER TOE

SAMUEL PARMAR

ANATOMICAL DEFINITION

Mallet toe involves distal interphalangeal joint.
Hammer toe involves proximal interphalangeal joint, sometimes involves hyperextension deformity of metatarsophalangeal joint.
Claw toe is hammer toe deformity of PIPJ and DIPJ with hyperextension deformity at the MTP joint.

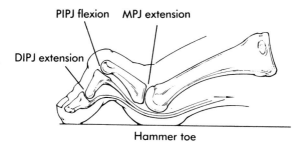

PIPJ flexion   MPJ extension

DIPJ extension

Hammer toe

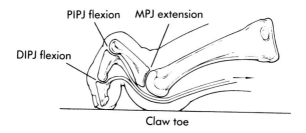

PIPJ flexion   MPJ extension

DIPJ flexion

Claw toe

PREVALENCE

Deformity develops slowly and is most common in women than in men.

Mallet Toe
- Usually develops secondary to tight shoes, status post hammer toe correction and inflammatory arthritis
- Pressure against the longest toe can cause plantar flexion at the distal interphalangeal joint.
- Tight flexor digitorum longus tendon can cause this deformity.
- Pediatric deformity associated with tight flexor tendon can result in curly toe.

Hammer Toe
- Constricting toe box
- Excessive pronation, hallux valgus deformity
- May be caused by muscle imbalance associated with neuromuscular disease
- Neuropathic disease such as diabetes mellitus
- Inflammatory disease such as rheumatoid arthritis
- Trauma

Claw Toe
- May be caused by imbalance between intrinsic and extrinsic musculatures
- Causes painful callus as metatarsal head is forced into a plantarflexed position, displacing fat pad distally, which can ultimately cause ulceration in severe cases

Biologic Etiology
- **Flexor stabilization:** Most common cause of contracted digits. Flexors overpower intrinsic muscle secondary to gaining mechanical advantage during late stance phase of gait
- **Flexor substitution:** Flexors overpower interossei caused by weakening of triceps surae muscles
- **Extensor substitution:** EDL gains mechanical advantage over lumbricals. It occurs secondary to excessive pull of triceps surae and EDL compensates by pulling harder in order to dorsiflex the ankle.

PHYSICAL EXAM

- Taut extensor digitorum longus tendons
- Evaluate for hyperkeratosis at distal tip of the toe, dorsal aspect of PIPJ caused by constant friction
- Evaluate for toe nail deformity
- Evaluate for interdigital hyperkeratosis
- Evaluate whether deformity is flexible versus rigid

RADIOGRAPHIC EXAM

- Obtain weight-bearing X-rays of affected foot
- Anterior-posterior view—evaluate for gun barrel sign, reduction in joint space at metatarsophalangeal joint and proximal interphalangeal joint and subluxation/dislocation of joint
- Lateral view—evaluate for severity of contracture

PROCEDURE SELECTION

Hammer Toe—Important to Evaluate Whether Deformity Is Rigid versus Flexible
- **Flexible deformity:** Flexor tendon transfer (Girdlestone-Taylor)
- **Rigid deformity:** Arthroplasty of head of proximal phalanx, soft tissue release at MTPJ and fixation with or without K-wire or implant
- Fusion of proximal interphalangeal joint using implant or K-wire fixation

Mallet Toe Correction
- Flexible—flexor tendon tenotomy
- Rigid—fusion of DIPJ or arthroplasty of middle phalanx and release of FDL tendon. Fixation via K-wire or implant

Deviated Toe at the Level of MTPJ
- Lengthening of extensor digitorum longus tendon if tendon is found to be taut
- Release of collateral ligaments, repair of plantar plate if indicated, and capsular reefing either laterally or medially to correct the deviation
- Chronic contracture of dorsal skin at the level of the metatarsophalangeal joint can be corrected via skin plasty (eg, V to Y technique, Z plasty).

5th Toe Deformity
Excision of skin wedge (usually planned preoperatively from distal medial to lateral proximal) and arthroplasty of head of proximal phalanx

SUGGESTED READINGS

Schrier JC, Keijsers NL, Matricali GA, Louwerens JW, Verheyen CC. Lesser toe PIP joint resection versus PIP joint fusion: a randomized clinical trial. *Foot Ankle Int.* 2016;37(6):569-575.

Wendelstein JA, Goger P, Bock P, Schuh R, Doz P, Trnka HJ. Bioabsorbable fixation screw for proximal interphalangeal arthrodesis of lesser toe deformities. *Foot Ankle Int.* 2017;38(9):1020-1025.

PLANTAR PLATE DYSFUNCTION

SCOTT T. BLEAZEY • ROSS M. SENTER

Plantar plate is the fibrocartilaginous continuation of the plantar fascia inserted onto the base of a proximal phalanx. Like the sesamoids of the hallux, it assists in the windlass mechanism during propulsion. Its fibers are oriented in a longitudinal, proximal to distal fashion. Upon dorsiflexion of the digits, during normal propulsion or secondary to trauma, the plantar plate is put under tension. In addition, the metatarsal heads and ground reactive forces provide additional compressive strain on the plantar plate. As the plantar plate is attached to the bases of the proximal phalanx, any digital dislocation, be it congenital, iatrogenic, or traumatic, can lead to plantar plate pathology. Most commonly affected is the second metatarsophalangeal joint as the second metatarsal is the longest. Additionally, the second metatarsal has unopposed lumbricals with no plantar interossei insertions.

ETIOLOGY

Abnormal forefoot loading
- Over-pronation during stance phase of gait
- Hallux abducto valgus
- Morton foot type (short first metatarsal compared with second)
- Trauma (hyperextension, excessive dorsiflexion at metatarsophalangeal joints)

CLASSIFICATION

Coughlin and Nery
- **Grade 0:** Plantar plate or capsular attenuation, and/or discoloration
- **Grade 1:** Transverse distal tear adjacent to insertion into proximal phalanx (<50%); medial/lateral/central area and/or midsubstance tear (<50%)
- **Grade 2:** Transverse distal tear (>50%); medial/lateral/central area and/or midsubstance tear (<50%)
- **Grade 3:** Transverse and/or longitudinal extensive tear (may involve collateral ligaments). Frequently, a distal transverse tear is also present.
- **Grade 4:** Extensive tear with button hole (dislocation); a combination of transverse and longitudinal tears; with an extensive tear, little plantar plate to repair

SIGNS AND SYMPTOMS

- Subluxation/dislocation of digits
- Pain in plantar forefoot
- Paresthesia
- Positive Lachman test (positive dorsal/plantar drawer test)

RADIOGRAPHIC FINDINGS (AP, LATERAL)

- Subluxation or dislocation of metatarsophalangeal joint
- Arthritic metatarsophalangeal joint
- Overlapping/underlapping digits
- Short first metatarsal
- Long second metatarsal
- Hallux abducto valgus

ULTRASOUND FINDINGS

- **Normal:** Slightly hyperechoic curved band
- **Abnormal:** Hypoechoic defect

MAGNETIC RESONANCE IMAGING FINDINGS

- Disruption of the plantar plate
- Increased signal intensity within and around plantar plate on T2-weighted imaging

CONSERVATIVE TREATMENT

- Taping/strapping digit in plantar flexion
- Offloading with padding, OTC versus custom orthoses
- Shoe gear modification
- NSAIDs
- Physical therapy—strengthening exercises
- Injections

SURGICAL MANAGEMENT

- With concomitant metatarsophalangeal joint jamming or excessively long metatarsal, a Weil osteotomy with snap-off screw fixation is recommended in conjunction with repair of plantar plate.
- Additional proximal interphalangeal joint arthrodesis may be required.

Type of plantar plate dysfunction:
- Attenuation—advancement of plantar plate with use of bone anchor
- Buttonhole/midsubstance longitudinal tear—side-to-side primary repair
- Partial tear—must complete tear of plantar plate, advance, and primary repair
- Complete tear—primary repair and advancement, possible flexor tendon augmentation

POSTOPERATIVE MANAGEMENT

- Rest
- Ice
- Elevation
- Compression
- Taping/strapping digit in plantar flexion
- NSAIDs

Partial weight bearing to heel versus CAM walker versus non–weight bearing
- Physical therapy

SUGGESTED READINGS

DeSandis B, Ellis SJ, Levitsky M. Rate of union after segmental midshaft shortening osteotomy of the lesser metatarsals. *Foot Ankle Int.* 2015;36(10):1190-1195.

Flint WW, Macias DM, Jastifer JR. Plantar plate repair for lesser metatarsophalangeal joint instability. *Foot Ankle Int.* 2017;38(3):234-242.

Watson TS, Reid DY, Frerichs TL. Dorsal approach for plantar plate repair with Weil osteotomy. *Foot Ankle Int.* 2014;35(7):730-739.

BUNIONETTES

SAMUEL PARMAR

DEFINITION

Painful prominence of lateral aspect of 5th metatarsal head

PHYSICAL EXAM

- Patient presents with pain and irritation at 5th met head prominence because of tight shoes, inflamed bursa, lateral keratosis, plantar keratosis.
- Foot type generally involves mild to severe flatfoot.
- Look for abducted 5th digit

RADIOGRAPH

- Radiographic evaluation involves obtaining three views of weight-bearing foot.
- **AP:** Fourth intermetatarsal angle normal range is 6.2 to 9.1 and symptomatic bunionettes according to McGlamry range between 8.7 and 10.8.
- **Lateral deviation angle:** Bisection of 5th metatarsal head and bisection of 5th metatarsal neck. Normal angle is 2.64

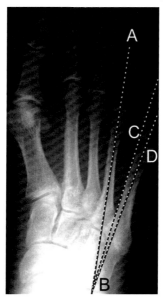

CONSERVATIVE TREATMENT

Range from wider shoes, padding and shaving of callosities caused secondary to prominent 5th met head

SURGICAL INTERVENTION

- Based on anatomical, radiographic symptoms of patient
- Lateral condylectomy where IM angle between 4th and 5th metatarsal is close to normal with presence of an enlarged lateral condyle. Condylectomy is resection of 1/4 to 1/3 lateral aspect of the 5th metatarsal head
- Distal 5th metatarsal osteotomies: Indicated to repair deformity arising from the osseous shape of the distal aspect of metatarsal
  - Chevron osteotomy—medial transposition of 5th metatarsal head

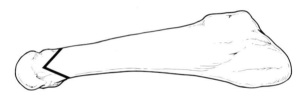

  - Hohmann osteotomy—transverse osteotomy with medial transposition of 5th metatarsal head with screw or K-wire fixation
- Midshaft osteotomy—increased lateral bowing
  - Closing lateral wedge osteotomy at level of metatarsal neck using screw or K-wire fixation

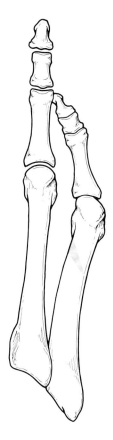

- Proximal 5th metatarsal osteotomy—enlarged fourth intermetatarsal angle and when deformity is too big to be corrected via distal osteotomy alone

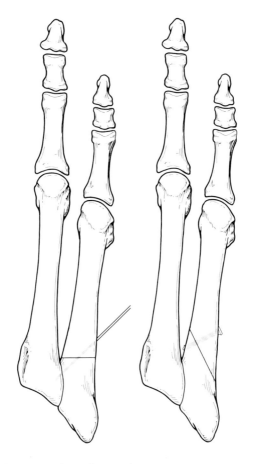

- Opening or closing base wedge osteotomy at metaphysis-diaphysis junction with screw fixation or plate

---

POST-OP CARE

- Distal osteotomy—immediate partial weight-bearing postoperatively with CAM Walker till radiographic union at osteotomy site, then transition to normal shoe gear as tolerated
- Middle and proximal osteotomy—immobilization in posterior splint or below knee cast till radiographic union of osteotomy site, transition to CAM Walker for 2 weeks and then weight bearing as tolerated in normal shoe gear

ABSOLUTE AND RELATIVE CONTRAINDICATION

Questionable vascular status, multiple comorbidities, noncompliant patient, immunocompromised patient

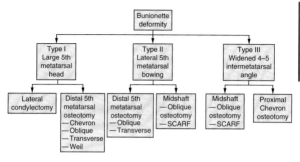

SUGGESTED READINGS

Coughlin MJ, Saltzman CL, Anderson RB. *Mann's Surgery of the Foot and Ankle*. 9th ed. Vol 1. Philadelphia, PA: Saunders/Elsevier; 2014.

McGlamry ED, Southerland JT. *McGlamry's Comprehensive Textbook of Foot and Ankle Surgery*. 4th ed. Vol 1. Philadelphia, PA: Wolters Kluwer Health/Lippincott Williams & Wilkins; 2013.

HANYA ALMUDALLAL

DEFINITIONS

- **Sesamoid:** Bony structure partially or totally embedded in a tendon
  Os peroneum: Within peroneus longus tendon at the level of the cuboid
  Os tibiale externum: Within posterior tibial tendon
  Os vesalianum: Within peroneus brevis tendon at the base of the 5th metatarsal
- **Accessory ossicles:** Supernumerary bones from unfused primary or secondary ossification sites
  Os trigonum: Posterior to talus
  Os intermetatarseum: Between 1st and 2nd metatarsal
  Os supranaviculare: Superior to navicular
  Os supratalare: Superior to distal talus
  Os calcaneus secundarius: Between anteromedial aspect of calcaneus, the cuboid, talar head, and tarsal navicular

1ST METATARSOPHALANGEAL JOINT SESAMOIDS

- Ellipsoidal synovial joint with capsule reinforced both medially and laterally by collateral ligaments
- The plantar plate acts as a stabilizer plantarly and fibular sesamoid attaches to the deep transverse metatarsal ligament. Tibial and fibular sesamoid bones are part of the 1st metatarsophalangeal joint and are located within the flexor hallucis brevis tendon.

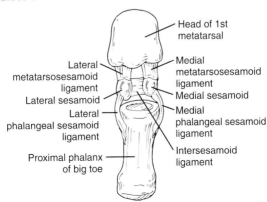

Head of 1st metatarsal

Lateral metatarsosesamoid ligament

Lateral sesamoid

Lateral phalangeal sesamoid ligament

Proximal phalanx of big toe

Medial metatarsosesamoid ligament

Medial sesamoid

Medial phalangeal sesamoid ligament

Intersesamoid ligament

FUNCTION

- Increase mechanical advantage of FHB tendon, assist in stabilization and load transmittance of 1st MPJ during gait (ie, propulsion)

CONSEQUENCES OF EXCISION

- Removal of tibial sesamoid may cause a hallux abducto valgus deformity.
- Removal of fibular sesamoid may cause a hallux varus deformity.
- Removal of both sesamoids may cause a hallux malleus deformity.

1ST METATARSOPHALANGEAL JOINT SPRAIN

- Usually from low-energy trauma, and sports related such as "turf toe," which is caused by hyperdorsiflexion of the 1st MPJ with the foot in plantar flexion
- **Clinical presentation:** Painful and swollen 1st MPJ, fracture may or may not be present

1ST METATARSOPHALANGEAL JOINT DISLOCATIONS/SESAMOID FRACTURE

- Rare, mostly occur from hyperdorsiflexion at 1st MTPJ with an axial load to the foot, or from trauma or motor vehicle accident
- **Clinical presentation:** Severe pain at the MTPJ, plantar ecchymosis
- **Jahss classification** (*McGlamry* 2012;2:1638):
  Type I: Hallux dislocated dorsally upon metatarsal head; sesamoids and intersesamoidal ligament remains intact. No separation or migration of sesamoids on X-ray. Treatment: Requires ORIF because of intact soft tissue attachments.
  Type IIA: Intersesamoidal ligament ruptured, sesamoids widely separated. Treatment: closed reduction.
  Type IIB: One sesamoid fractures transversely (usually medial), with distal fragment of fracture displacing distally on X-ray. No widening between sesamoids noted. Treatment: closed reduction.
  Type IIC: Combination of Type IIA and Type IIB. Fracture of sesamoid as well as sesamoidal widening may be present. Treatment: closed reduction.

BIPARTITE SESAMOID

- Normal variant. 10% of population has bipartite sesamoid. Of these, 25% will have it bilaterally (*Insights Imaging* 2013;4(5):581-593).
- Bone edges will be smooth and distinct, not jagged and irregular like a fractured sesamoid.
- Tibial sesamoid is more likely to be bipartite than fibular sesamoid.
- Always get bilateral X-ray to rule out fracture.

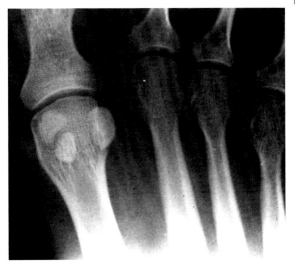

SESAMOID FRACTURE

- Must differentiate between fracture and bipartite sesamoid
- **Imaging:** X-ray, CT, bone scan, MRI
- Acute fracture on MRI shows increased signal intensity on T2 images.
- **Conservative therapy:** Rest, ice, compression, elevation, off-loading
- **Surgical treatment:** Partial or complete excision

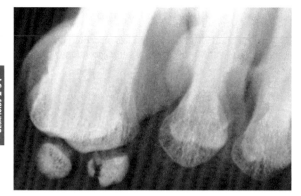

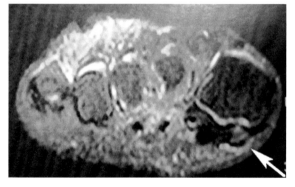

SESAMOIDITIS

- When tendon surrounding sesamoid becomes inflamed. Common in runners and dancers.
- **Clinical presentation:** Pain and swelling at plantar 1st MPJ, particularly while walking. MRI may be helpful.
- **Treatment:** Conservative therapy RICE and shoe modification; if symptoms persist, then may consider surgical removal of sesamoid.

Images in this chapter from Southerland JT, Vickers DF, Boberg JS. *McGlamry's Comprehensive Textbook of Foot and Ankle Surgery*. 4th ed. Philadelphia, PA: Lippincott Williams & Wilkins; 2013.

NAIL DISORDERS

HANYA ALMUDALLAL

NAIL ANATOMY

- **Eponychium:** Cuticle, posterior nail fold
- **Hyponychium:** Distal nail groove
- **Ungual labia:** Medial and lateral nail fold

NAIL PATHOLOGY

- **Anonychia:** Absence of nail, lack of development
- **Beau lines:** Horizontal depression across nail plate caused by arrest of nail growth. Stressful event, such as MI, PE, or high fever, can be the cause.
- **Blue nails:** May be caused by exposure to silver nitrate, drugs (minocycline, antimalarial), Wilson disease, iron metabolism disorder
- **Brown nail:** Occurs with Addison disease, hemochromatosis, arsenic intoxication, malignant melanoma, Nelson syndrome
- **Dystrophic nail:** Caused by trauma or malnutrition
- **Gray nail/lunula:** Caused by prolonged ingestion or absorption of silver nitrate
- **Green nail:** Pseudomonas infection
- **Hapalonychia:** Pliable, thin nail plate caused by endocrine disorders or hyperhidrosis
- **Herpetic Whitlow:** Severe herpetic viral infection of distal phalanx. Erythematous streaking of extremity and prominent lymph nodes may also be noted.
- **Clubbing:** Occurs in pulmonary disease (metastatic cancer, bronchiectasis, mesothelioma), cardiac disease (bacterial endocarditis, cyanotic heart disease), or GI disease (ulcerative colitis and hepatic cirrhosis). Considered "clubbed" when Lovibond angle between nail plate and proximal nail fold is >180°
- **Koilonychia (Spoon nail):** Long-standing iron deficiency anemia or Plummer-Vinson syndrome (triad of koilonychias, dysphagia, and glossitis)
- **Leukonychia:** White spots (punctata) or striata
- **Lindsay nails:** Distal half is pink/brown and the proximal half of nail is dull/white. Caused by liver disease and azotemia
- **Macronychia:** Abnormally large nail
- **Mees lines:** Single transverse white band seen with arsenic poisoning

- **Melanonychia:** Pigmented longitudinal bands in the nails. May be a sign of malignant melanoma or a normal variant in darker-skinned individuals
- **Micronychia:** Abnormally small nail
- **Muehrcke nails:** Paired narrow horizontal white bands, separated by normal color. Associated with hypoalbuminemia from nephrotic syndrome
- **Onychatrophia:** Atrophy of nail
- **Onychauxic:** Hypertrophy of nail
- **Onychia:** Inflammation of nail matrix
- **Onychoclasis:** Breaking of nail
- **Onychocryptosis:** Ingrowing nail
- **Onychogryphosis:** Hypertrophic nail curled distally over digit
- **Onychoheterotopia:** Abnormal location of nail growth because of displaced matrix material
- **Onychomadesis:** Separation of nail plate from nail bed beginning proximally and progressing distally
- **Onychomalacia:** Soft nail
- **Onychomycosis:** Fungal nail, most commonly caused by *Trichophyton rubrum*
- **Onychophosis:** Callus in nail groove
- **Onychopunctata:** Pitting of the nails associated with psoriasis, alopecia areata, and lichen planus
- **Onychorrhexis:** Brittle nails because of lack of hydration <16%. Normal nail hydration 16% to 30%
- **Onychoschizia:** Splitting of nail plate into layers
- **Paronychia:** Inflammation of nail folds/tissue
- **Pterygium:** Overgrowth of cuticle. Associated with lichen planus, scleroderma, and dermatomyositis
- **Red lunula:** Caused by right-sided CHF
- **Splinter hemorrhages:** Seen in subacute bacterial endocarditis and trichinosis (from inadequately cooked meat infected with *Trichinella spiralis*)
- **Subungual exostosis:** Benign bony lesion protrudes from dorsal surface of distal phalanx, causing the nail plate to be deformed. Common in hallux
- **Subungual hematoma:** Blood trapped between nail plate and nail bed from acute trauma (ie, dropping something on toe). Increased pressure under the nail may lead to necrosis of tissue.
- **Telangiectatic posterior nail fold:** Proximal nail fold is dilated. Associated with connective tissue disorders like lupus and dermatomyositis

- **Terry nails:** Proximal two-thirds of nail plate is white, distal one-third is red. Associated with hypoalbuminemia with hepatic cirrhosis
- **Yellow nail syndrome:** Slow-growing, thick, curved nail with onycholysis. Associated with pulmonary disease and lymphedema (*Pocket Podiatrics* 3:316-319)

KERATOTIC ABNORMALITIES

Epidermis
- **Stratum corneum:** Outermost layer of epidermis, composed of dry, flattened, anuclear, and dead skin cells that flake off the body
- **Stratum lucidum:** Clear, translucent layer of epidermis
- **Stratum granulosum:** Cytoplasm with keratohyalin granules, several cell layers thick
- **Stratum spinosum:** Intercellular bridges give the cells a spiny appearance, several cell layers thick
- **Basement membrane (stratum germinativum, basal layer):** Deepest layer of epidermis, composed of single layer of proliferating cells that migrate slowly upward to the stratum corneum

Dermis
Dense connective tissue forming bulk of skin. Contains nerves, blood vessels, lymphatic vessels, and hair follicles
- **Reticular layer:** Lower two-thirds of dermis. Contains Pacinian corpuscles
- **Papillary layer:** Upper one-third of dermis. Contains Meissner corpuscles
- **Subcutaneous tissue (hypodermis):** Fatty connective tissue

Additional Cells
- **Melanocytes:** Among the basal cells, produce melanin which absorbs and is activated by UV light and protects tissue
- **Langerhans cells:** Within epidermis, function as macrophages of skin to fight infection

Primary Keratotic Lesions
- **Macule:** Flat, circumscribed lesion <1 cm in diameter, not raised
- **Patch:** Flat lesion, >1 cm in diameter
- **Papule:** Circumscribed, solid and elevated lesion <1 cm in diameter
- **Plaque:** Circumscribed and elevated lesion >1 cm in diameter

- **Nodule:** Circumscribed solid elevated lesion <1 cm with element of depth (unlike papule)
- **Tumor:** Circumscribed solid elevated lesion >1 cm with element of depth (unlike plaque)
- **Vesicle:** Fluid-filled elevated lesion <0.5 cm in diameter
- **Bulla:** Fluid-filled elevated lesion >0.5 cm in diameter
- **Cyst:** Noninfected deep collection of material surrounded by histologically definable wall
- **Burrow:** Intraepidermal tunneling usually caused by insects or parasites
- **Wheal (hives):** Well-circumscribed, elevated lesion that appears and then disappears rapidly
- **Pustule:** Vesicle or bulla containing purulent fluid (*Pocket Podiatrics* 3:260)

Secondary Keratotic Lesions
- **Scaling:** Exfoliative condition marked by flaking lamination of epidermis
- **Excoriation:** Scratch marks seen associated with pruritis
- **Lichenification:** Thickening of skin with a leathery appearance and associated hyperpigmentation. Can be caused by excessive scratching/rubbing
- **Erosion:** Deep excoriations in epidermis, but dermis is not affected. Does not cause scarring
- **Ulcer:** Deep epidermal defect in which dermis is affected. May cause scarring
- **Crust:** Dried areas of serum, blood, and pus
- **Fissure:** Deep linear, epidermal cracks found in areas of dry or thickened skin
- **Scar:** Formation of fibrous connective tissue replacing dermis, which has been lost because of trauma or iatrogenic cause
- **Maceration:** Overly white appearance of epidermis because of overhydration

Dermatitis
- **Contact dermatitis:** Caused by contact with environmental substances causing inflammation of epidermis and dermis
  Classic examples: Poison ivy, nickel in jewelry, shoe gear
  Irritation contact dermatitis: Nonimmunologic, single exposure may cause reaction (ie, detergents).
  Allergic contact dermatitis: Acquired immunologic response, requires repeat exposure (ie, poison ivy)
  Presentation: Irregular, poorly demarcated patches of erythema and edema with vesicles and erosions exuding serum and crust

- **Urticaria:** Allergic reaction causing pruritic wheals to erupt within 24 hours of allergen exposure
  May be caused by food, drugs, and parasites
  May cause anaphylaxis if reaction is severe
- **Lichen simplex chronicus (neurodermatitis):** Circumscribed area of lichenification as a result of repetitive scratching or rubbing of skin
- **Dyshidrotic eczematous dermatitis (dyshidrosis):** Vesicular type of eczema with associated pruritis, but not associated with hyperhidrosis
  Bullous form: Pompholyx
  Caused by: Emotional stress, ingestion of nickel, cobalt, or chromium
  Presentation: Sides of soles of feet with small deep-seated vesicles in clusters
- **Seborrheic dermatitis:** Chronic inflammatory disorder characterized by scaling and redness, usually worse in winter
  Presentation: Erythematous patches with flaking, white scales. Commonly located in the scalp, eyebrows, beard, central back, but may also present on feet

Bacterial Infections
- **Impetigo:** Contagious skin infection, most commonly caused by *Staphylococcus aureus*
  Presentation: Red rash with small blisters that drain fluid and form a honey-colored crust
- **Pitted keratolysis:** Superficial pitting of stratum corneum on soles of feet
  Presentation: Lesion to plantar foot appearing "moth eaten"
  Caused by keratolytic enzymes of bacteria *Corynebacterium* or *Micrococcus sedentarius*, commonly associated with hyperhidrosis or bromohidrosis
- **Erythrasma:** Bacterial infection of intertriginous areas of body (ie, between toes)
  More common in warm, humid climates and in diabetics
  Caused by *Corynebacterium minutissimum* or as a secondary infection of *Tinea pedis*
  May use Wood lamp to differentiate between fungal and bacterial cause: (+) coral red under Wood lamp indicates bacterial cause
  Presentation: Scaling, fissuring and macerated, most commonly between the 3rd and 4th digits

Fungal Skin Infections

- **Tinea pedis (Athlete's foot):** Cutaneous mycosis, does not become systemic, but may elicit an immune response

  Causes:

  Microsporum: Infects skin and hair. Fluoresces green under UV light. Rarely causes T. Pedis.

  Epidermophyton floccosum: Infects skin and nail. Third most common cause of T. Pedis

  Trichophyton mentagrophytes: Vesicular lesions to plantar skin or may be intertriginous, especially to 3rd interspace. Maceration, scaling, and fissuring with pruritis and malodor. This is the second most common cause of T. Pedis.

  Trichophyton rubrum: Infects skin, hair, and nails. Most common cause of T. Pedis. Moccasin-like distribution on plantar and sides of foot, may also present with intertriginous form.

NERVE DISORDERS

CARL M. JEAN • ALEKSANDR EMEREL

BASIC (PERIPHERAL) NERVE ANATOMY

- **Epineurium:** The outermost layer of dense irregular connective tissue surrounding a peripheral nerve
- **Perineurium:** The connective tissue sheath surrounding each bundle of nerve fibers (fascicle) in a peripheral nerve
- **Endoneurium:** Layer of delicate connective tissue around the myelin sheath of each myelinated nerve fiber
- **Schwann cell:** Any of the cells that surround the axons of the peripheral nerves, forming the myelin sheath of myelinated nerve fibers and providing support for non-myelinated nerve fibers
- **Nodes of Ranvier:** Periodic gap in the insulating sheath (myelin) on the axon of certain neurons that serves to facilitate the rapid conduction of nerve impulses. Occur at approximately 1-mm intervals

EVIDENCE-BASED ALGORITHMS

- **Tinel sign:** Sign of an irritated nerve. Positive when lightly percussing over the nerve elicits a sensation of tingling, or "pins and needles," in the distribution of the nerve
- **Valleix sign:** Proximal radiation of pain and paresthesia along the neuraxis on percussion at the point of nerve injury
- Nerve blocks
- Two-point discrimination
- Monofilament testing (loss of touch-pressure of 10 kg/cm^2)
- **NCV/EMG:** NCV measures sensory nerves in an antidromic way and can suggest nerve entrapment or demyelinating disease; EMG can assess denervation of muscle based on skeletal muscle electrical activity. Measured by inserting needle
- Ancillary devices (ie, AcroVal: PSSD, AcroGrip, AcroPinch)

TYPES OF NERVE INJURIES

- Traction neuritis (scarring and adhesions)
- Compression or entrapment of the nerve
- Partially transected nerve
- Fully transected nerve
- Stump neuroma
- Neuroma-in-continuity
- Indeterminate pathology and ideology

GENERAL SURGICAL CONSIDERATIONS

NERVE DISORDERS 3-2

- Patient age
- Patient health status/comorbidities
- Age of injury
- Mechanism of injury
- Extent of nerve tissue damage
- Finding healthy nerve ends
- Tension at the repair site
- Best method in bridging the gap
- Barriers to control ingrowth and axonal escape
- Scarring and entrapment
- Vascularity of the nerve and surrounding tissue
- Use of technologies including nerve connectors/conduits, nerve wraps, and nerve allograft

EVIDENCE-BASED EVOLUTION OF NERVE REPAIR/ OTHER CONSIDERATIONS

- **Reconstructive technique:** Primary versus connector-assisted versus allograft versus autograft
- **Coaptation site:** Connector-assisted coaptation versus suture alone
- **Repair stable with ROM:** Ensure a mechanically stable repair, under ROM
- **Minimizing collateral sprouting/optimize neurotropism:** Nerve connectors/protectors, bury in muscle or bone or fat
- Consider use of local muscle flaps for coverage/addition of structural support following nerve repair

COMMON NERVE CONDITIONS OF THE FOOT

Interdigital Neuroma
- Entrapment or neuritis of a common digital nerve
- Most often found in the 3rd interspace between the 3rd and 4th metatarsal heads as described by Morton in 1876
- Eight to 10 times more common in women due to hyperextension of MTP joints caused by footwear
- Located below the DTML

Physical Exam
- +Mulder's click
- +Lateral squeeze test

Imaging

- **MRI:** Shows inflammation around neuroma on T2-weighted images
- **Ultrasound:** Shows a noncompressible, hypoechoic interdigital mass

Etiology

Anatomic	Traumatic	Extrinsic
• The common digital nerve to the 3rd interspace has increased thickness and is more subject to neuroma formation • Mobility of the medial three rays and lateral two rays causes increased mobility in the third web space	• Fall from height or crush injury • Previous metatarsal fracture	• Soft tissue mass above or below the DTML • Bursitis • Thickened DTML • Plantar plate degeneration

Conservative Treatment

- Wider shoes, strapping, metatarsal support
- Injection of the interspace, anti-inflammatories

Surgical Treatment

- Excision of the nerve via dorsal or plantar approach
- **Dorsal approach:** Violates DTML, better scar formation
- **Plantar approach:** Does not violate DTML, potential for scar formation
- Revisional surgery or recurrent neuromas should be carried out through plantar approach.

FOOT DROP

- Inability to DF the ankle
- Steppage gait with equinovarus deformity
- Damage to the CPN or paralysis of anterior muscle group
- MC cause is L4/L5 radiculopathy from disc herniation.
- Second MC cause is CFN neuropathy.

Physical Exam
- Babinski reflex
- Hoffmann test

Etiology

Neurologic	Trauma	Systemic
• Peroneal nerve injury	• Fibular fracture	• Diabetes
• Sciatic nerve injury	• Compartment syndrome	• Alcoholism
• Spinal cord lesions	• Rupture of tibialis anterior tendon	• Polio
• Cauda equina syndrome		• CMT
• Stroke		• Muscular dystrophy
• TIA		

Studies
- **X-rays:** Rule out trauma, Charcot
- **MRI:** Rule out tumor, compressive lesion, tendon ruptures
- **NCV/EMG:** Neuropathic origins

Conservative Treatment
- Sympathetic block
- **Bracing:** AFO
- PT
- Nerve stimulator

Surgical Treatment
- Posterior tibial tendon transfer
- Peroneus longus tendon transfer
- Bridle procedure
- Arthrodesis (ankle and/or STJ) when rigid or involves neurologic symptoms

---

BAXTER'S NEURITIS

- **Baxter's nerve:** First branch of the lateral plantar nerve. It is another name for the inferior calcaneal nerve, which runs beneath the heel bone. Believed to innervate periosteum of the heel
- Baxter's neuritis or Baxter's nerve entrapment may cause heel pain, which can be confused with plantar fasciitis.

Predisposing Factors
- Muscle hypertrophy (ie, abductor hallux muscle, quadratus plantae)
- Obesity
- Hyperpronated foot
- Flatfoot
- Plantar calcaneal spur
- Plantar fasciitis
- Seronegative spondyloarthropathies
- Presents mostly between 25 and 50 years of age

Radiographic (MRI) Features

- **Acute phase of muscle denervation:** Affected region shows decreased signal intensity on T1 and increased signal intensity on T2 with fat saturation due to increased extracellular water content and decreased muscle fiber volume of the involved muscles innervated by the inferior calcaneal nerve.
- **Chronic phase of muscle denervation:** Signs of amyotrophy or fatty degeneration of the abductor digiti minimi muscle and less commonly of the flexor digitorum brevis and the quadratus plantae muscles

Clinical Presentation

- No specific test, diagnosed clinically
- Can use small amount of injected lidocaine with ultrasound guidance: Numbness of the heel is the strong evidence for Baxter's neuritis
- Heel pain with maximal tenderness over the course of the inferior calcaneal nerve (plantar medial foot and anterior to the medial aspect of the calcaneus)
- Paresthesia with motor weakness of the abductor digit minimi muscle
- No associated cutaneous sensory deficit
- Unlike plantar fasciitis that is worse after rest or getting out of bed, Baxter's neuritis may continue after one is off the feet. Burning or sharp shooting pain is often present. Pain occasionally located at the edges of the heel, either inner or outer.

Treatment

- Prescribed stretches, physical therapy, taping of the heel to control uncontrollable motions, NSAIDs, custom orthotics
- Chemical neurolysis, radiofrequency ablation
- Surgical release of the nerve

TARSAL TUNNEL SYNDROME

- Entrapment neuropathy involving the posterior tibial nerve within the tarsal canal behind the medial malleolus
- Flexor retinaculum covers the posterior tibial, flexor digitorum longus, and flexor hallucis longus tendons. It also covers the posterior tibial artery, vein, and posterior tibial nerve.
- PT nerve has three terminal branches: Medial plantar, lateral plantar, and medial calcaneal.
- Pain is described as burning, numbing, tingling relieved by rest and aggravated by activity.

Physical Exam
- Diffuse pain along medial ankle and medial plantar foot
- +**Tinel sign:** Percussion of the nerve generates radiation of pain distally along the course of the nerve.
- +**Valleix sign:** Percussion of the nerve generates radiation of pain proximally along the course of the nerve.

Studies
- **MRI/US:** to rule out (r/o) space-occupying mass
- **Nerve conduction studies:** to rule out neuropathies or proximal nerve lesions

Etiology

- **Idiopathic:** most common
- Traumatic
- Varicosities
- Space-occupying mass
- Heel varus
- Fibrosis
- Diabetes
- Obesity

Conservative Treatment
- Only indicated if no presence of space-occupying lesion
- NSAIDs, vitamin B_6, tricyclic antidepressants, gabapentin
- Topical agents like lidocaine or capsaicin
- Injection with steroid
- Immobilization with CAM walker
- Physical therapy

Surgical Treatment
- Performed with or without a tourniquet
- Incision performed from medial aspect of medial malleolus to top of the TN joint
- The flexor retinaculum is released followed by the MPN and the LPN.
- The flexor retinaculum is not re-approximated during closure.
- Tarsal tunnel release should be considered as a prophylactic procedure when performing varus to valgus corrections:
  - Tibial varum deformity (angular correction)
  - Dwyer osteotomy
  - Lateral calcaneal displacement osteotomy
  - Other deformities: Procurvatum to recurvatum

SUGGESTED READING

Baxter DE, Pfeffer GB. Treatment of chronic heel pain by surgical release of the first branch of the lateral plantar nerve. *Clin Orthop Relat Res.* 1992;(279):229-236.

Cimino WR. Tarsal tunnel syndrome: review of the literature. *Foot Ankle Int.* 1990;11(1):47-52.

PLANTAR HEEL PAIN

KONSTANTIN AGARUNOV • CORY P. CLEMENT • ROCK C. J. POSITANO •
RONALD M. GUBERMAN • ROCK G. POSITANO

BIOMECHANICAL/MECHANICAL

- A self-limiting condition is present in up to 15% of adults that may have a prolonged course w/numerous nomenclature based on suspected etiology: Plantar fasciitis, plantar fasciosis, plantar fascialgia, calcaneodynia, heel spur syndrome, plantar fascia degeneration, superficial or deep surface partial tearing of the plantar fascia, plantar fibroma (*J Am Podiatric Med Assoc* 2015;105(2))
- **Symptoms:** Pain at plantar heel and/or proximal medial arch with first step in the morning and with ambulation after periods of rest (poststatic dyskinesia), could quell w/activity and then relapse, pain w/prolonged standing, symptoms exacerbated by walking barefoot or in flat/unsupportive shoegear
- **Etiology:** Traction of plantar fascia and soft tissues at insertion to inferior calcaneus leading to microtears and degeneration, secondary to biomechanical instability or repetitive microtrauma, correlation w/obesity/high BMI, presence of atrophied plantar fat pad, rule out a contour or non-contour plantar fascia deforming plantar fibroma
- **Diagnostic evaluation:** Localized edema at plantar-medial heel; pain on palpation at central plantar/plantar-medial heel, at medial calcaneal tubercle, and at proximal medial and/or central band of plantar fascia; passive extension of toes could elicit or exacerbate symptoms by engaging windlass mechanism and placing tension on the fascia; presence of biomechanical imbalances such as excessively pronated or cavus foot type, limited ankle dorsiflexion w/Achilles tendon contracture, tibial varum, limb length discrepancy, plantar fibroma pain is sudden and may occur after vigorous exercise or with use of a different shoe than is customary. Check the palmar aspect of the hands for Dupuytren contracture. Bilateral heel pain should be worked up for seronegative arthritis and other rheumatologic conditions. Check for the presence of psoriasis as psoriatic arthritis may be present. Rheumatoid blood profile should include screening for HLA-B27 antigen. Check for handedness (right vs left)

Radiographs may show inferior calcaneal spur if symptoms present >6 months, which does not necessarily correlate w/ presence or severity of symptoms. Diagnostic ultrasound best visualizes the presence of plantar fibroma and plantar fascia superficial and deep partial tearing. Ultrasound may also exhibit thickened plantar aponeurosis.

- **Initial treatment:** Daily stretching of Achilles tendon and plantar fascia, RICE therapy, manual massage, padding and strapping, OTC foot orthoses including heel lifts and heel cups, NSAIDs (PO/topical), corticosteroid injection into point of maximum tenderness, change in shoegear, avoidance of barefoot walking, weight loss
- **Treatment of recalcitrant pain:** Continuation of prior treatment protocol, subsequent corticosteroid injections (multiple injections may cause plantar fascial rupture or fat pad atrophy) (*Foot Ankle Int* 1998;19(2):91), custom foot orthoses, physical therapy, night splints, immobilization/casting or pneumatic walking boot, PRP injection (*Foot Ankle Int* 2014;35(4):313), Botox injection, ESWT
- Surgical intervention indicated in patients unresponsive to 6 or more months of conservative therapy. Includes percutaneous radiofrequency coblation, open plantar fasciotomy/fasciectomy w/ or w/o heel spur resection, minimally invasive and endoscopic fasciotomy (*J Foot Ankle Surg* 2010;49:S1)

NEUROGENIC

- **Symptoms:** Similar to and may occur concomitantly w/mechanical heel pain, usually unilateral, exacerbated by increased activity w/ or w/o correlation to poststatic state, local or regional burning, tingling, or numbness, "pins and needles," electric- or shooting-type pain, which may radiate distally or originate proximally from the lower back, traveling inferiorly to the posterior thigh, leg, or heel
- **Etiology:** Local or proximal nerve impingement involving either the first branch of lateral plantar nerve (mixed sensory/motor branch to abductor digiti minimi muscle, also named Baxter nerve, inferior calcaneal nerve), tibial nerve or its branches within the tarsal tunnel, medial calcaneal nerve, spinal nerve compression or sciatica with radiating pain, previous surgery or trauma to heel or ankle causing neuritis. Bilateral presentation may indicate systemic polyneuropathy (DM, alcoholism, chemotherapy).
- **Diagnostic evaluation:** HPI yields unsuccessful prior conservative treatment for suspected or associated mechanical heel pain. Also persistently elevated blood sugar, history of alcoholism, or prior course of chemo- or radiotherapy can indicate local signs of systemic disease. Passive dorsiflexion

of the ankle coupled w/heel eversion and extension of toes could elicit symptoms (*J Bone Joint Surg Am* 2001;83-A(12): 1835); compression or percussion of nerve at tarsal tunnel or plantar/medial heel may be associated w/proximal or distal radiating pain (+Valleix, Tinel signs) distinct from medial calcaneal tubercle pain, decreased sharp/dull, vibratory, and proprioceptive sensation; EMG/NCV studies to evaluate for tarsal tunnel syndrome might exhibit decreased velocities, excessive pronation on biomechanical exam causing tension on tibial nerve within tarsal tunnel, straight leg raise to elicit sciatic nerve pain radiating to heel. MRI warranted for evaluation of tarsal tunnel-occupying lesions (varicosities, ganglions) or muscle atrophy from prolonged denervation. MRI of lumbosacral spine to rule out L4, L5 and S1 pathology

- **Treatment:** Conservative treatment similar to that for mechanical heel pain, orthoses, offloading, corticosteroid injections for neuritis, physical therapy, vitamin B supplementation. Referral to neurology for proximal disease such as sciatica or radiculopathy, prior cancer treatment or alcoholism. Referral to PCP or endocrinology for neuropathy caused by uncontrolled DM
- Surgical correction involves release of entrapped nerves and structures within the tarsal tunnel w/ or w/o isolated decompression of first branch of lateral plantar nerve (*Am Fam Physician* 1999;59(8):2200; *Man Ther* 2008;13(2):103).

ARTHRITIC

- **Symptoms:** Plantar heel pain in poststatic setting but often lasting an hour or longer, often in conjunction w/multiple symmetrical or asymmetrical joint pains and significant stiffness, especially in the morning, symptoms can be migratory, various skin lesions, burning upon urination, eye irritation, back pain
- **Etiology:** Local manifestation of systemic disease, such as rheumatoid arthritis, and seronegative arthropathies, such as psoriatic arthritis, ankylosing spondylitis, diffuse idiopathic skeletal hyperostosis (DISH), Reiter syndrome (reactive arthritis), systemic lupus erythematosus, Paget disease of bone, gout, fibromyalgia
- **Diagnostic evaluation:** Thorough PMH and HPI paramount to diagnosis including previous treatment and consultation, unlike self-limiting nature of mechanical heel pain symptoms often recur despite prolonged conservative management, physical exam can yield symmetric pain, swelling, and stiffness

in the joints of the feet and hands, as well as fibular deviation of the digits in the setting of rheumatoid arthritis, asymmetrical involvement w/psoriatic arthritis, presence of tophi in pedal joints, lab work such as CBC, rheumatoid profile, and CMP will yield systemic abnormalities not present in mechanical or neurogenic heel pain. Joint aspiration and analysis of affected joints may differentiate inflammatory or infectious from noninflammatory process. Radiographs exhibit inferior spurring with resorption of spur with psoriatic arthritis, fluffy periostitis w/Reiter syndrome, or calcification/ossification of plantar fascia, cortical thickening w/Paget disease, bony erosions at plantar calcaneus can occur w/gout, psoriatic arthritis, rheumatoid and other arthritic processes (*Radiographics* 1991;11(3):415). Advanced imaging such as MRI or CT is helpful in differentiating etiology and extent of involvement.

- **Treatment:** Previously mentioned conservative treatment, systemic corticosteroids, DMARDs, accompanied by prompt referral to rheumatology, dermatology, or other appropriate clinical specialty
- Surgical management reserved for cases recalcitrant to systemic treatment by medical subspecialty and geared toward relieving symptomatology

TRAUMATIC

- **Symptoms:** Diffuse, poorly localized pain
- **Etiology:** Memorable traumatic event such as fall from height or MVA; intense physical activity, especially w/repetitive floor contact, such as running, stress/extra- or intra-articular (subtalar joint posterior facet) calcaneal body fracture, fracture of inferior spur, anterior process, or sustentaculum tali; posttraumatic arthritis from prior injury; acute plantar fascial rupture (especially w/previous multiple corticosteroid injections)
- **Diagnostic evaluation:** Plantar ecchymosis, pain elicited w/side-to-side compression of calcaneus, often diffuse over entire heel as opposed to a discrete trigger point. Radiographs (can be negative within 7-14 days of sustained stress fracture) demonstrate sclerosis, disruption of trabecular pattern, or overt fracture; CT to evaluate articular surfaces of subtalar joint. MRI, bone scan if plain film is negative or if contraindication to MRI, such as metal implant, is present
- **Treatment:** Immobilization, splinting, casting, non–weight bearing, physical therapy
- Surgery warranted for displaced and/or intra-articular fractures consisting of ORIF, percutaneous pinning, or joint fusion

OTHER CAUSES

- **Neoplasm:** Benign or malignant calcaneal tumor, calcaneus is most vascular bone and most common site of primary bone tumor as well as metastasis in the foot, may have insidious course. Radiographs may demonstrate expansile single or lobulated lesion, lytic or blastic changes. DDX includes solitary/unicameral/aneurismal/hemorrhagic bone cyst, giant cell tumor, osteoblastoma, intraosseous lipoma, fibrous dysplasia, indicating referral to hematology/oncology or orthopedic oncology.
- **Apophysitis:** Sever disease, unilateral or bilateral pain caused by soft tissue traction on an open calcaneal growth plate in adolescents, exacerbated w/physical activity such as sports. Radiographs demonstrate sclerosis of calcaneal apophysis, treated by immobilization, non–weight bearing, orthoses, physical therapy (*J Pediatr Orthop* 1987;7(1):34).
- **Infection:** Soft tissue infection or osteomyelitis, symptoms include erythema and edema, which is localized or w/proximal extension, often history of puncture wound to heel. If open wound present, may be accompanied by purulent drainage, malodor, possibly hematogenous spread, especially in pediatrics. Radiographs may demonstrate soft tissue emphysema and/or osteolytic changes. Treat w/incision and drainage if abscess, PO or IV antibiotics depending on severity
- **Charcot neuroarthropathy:** Symptoms include diffuse edema and/or erythema, present in uncontrolled diabetes, chronic alcoholism. Radiographs demonstrate gross destruction of bone and joints, treated w/immobilization and strict non–weight bearing
- **Vascular:** Sharp, often diffuse pain, intermittent or constant, can be exacerbated by ambulation or other physical activity, present in smokers, uncontrolled diabetes, due to calcification, stenosis, or occlusion of blood vessels. Physical exam yields delayed capillary refill to digits, faint or absent pedal, popliteal pulses, may be accompanied by hyperesthesia and dusky discoloration of pedal skin and nail beds. Diagnosis confirmed by ABI/PVR/TCPO$_2$. Radiographs may demonstrate calcified vessels. May benefit from oral venodilator such as cilostazol. Referral to vascular surgery for endovascular intervention, such as angioplasty w/ or w/o stenting, or open intervention, such as bypass

JILLIAN M. KAZLEY • MATTHEW R. DICAPRIO

INFECTIONS

Osteomyelitis: Infection of the bone causing destruction and apposition of new bone (*Lancet* 2004;364:36; *Clin Ortho Relat Res* 2003;414:7)

- **Risk factors:** Trauma, immunocompromised, poor vascularity, DM
- **Mechanism:** Hematogenous, contiguous-focus (trauma, wounds, poor vascularity), direct inoculation via penetrating injuries, previous surgeries
- **Workup:** WBC, ESR, CRP, blood cx, bone cx/biopsy
  - **WBC:** Elevated in acute osteo; may be normal in chronic cases
  - **ESR, CRP:** Elevated in both acute and chronic osteo
  - CRP is most sensitive to monitor treatment
  - **Blood cx:** dx of hematogenous osteo, often negative soon after initiation of abx
  - **Bone cx/biopsy:** Gold standard for abx-guided therapy, sinus tract/exposed bone cx not recommended due to unreliability
- **Imaging:** XR only apparent after 30% bone loss, radiolucent region surrounded by sclerosis
  - **Sequestrum:** Devitalized bone that serves as nidus for infection
  - **Involucrum:** New bone formation about areas of bone necrosis
  - **CT:** Helpful for surgical planning
  - **MRI:** Highly sensitive and specific, helps to differentiate soft tissue and bone involvement

Cierny Classification	
Location	**Host**
I–Medullary	A–Normal
II–Superficial	B–Compromised
III–Localized	C–Treatment is more dangerous than infection
IV–Diffuse	

- **Timing:** Acute < 2 weeks, subacute 2 to 6 weeks, chronic > 6 weeks
- **Treatment:** Abx–initial therapy for 4 to 6 weeks
  Irrigation and debridement, then organism-targeted abx
  Failure of initial therapy, abx therapy, leads to more chronic osteo with abscess or draining sinus tract

Brodie abscess: Subacute osteomyelitis bone
- **Background:** Most common in metaphyseal bone of children via hematogenous seeding

  May appear at the distal tibia, talus, or the apophysis of the calcaneus. Risk factors: local trauma or bacteremia
- **Presentation:** Deep pain that is often worse at night and relieved with rest, or asymptotic found incidentally
- **Imaging/Dx:** XR: abscess appears as a circular lucency surrounded by a zone of sclerosis.
- **Treatment:** Aspiration: helps to guide abx if organism is identified by cx, abx should help improve clinically in 48 hours continue 4 to 6 weeks

  Surgical evacuation and curettage that may be packed with abx-impregnated bone cement if the cavity is large

Puncture wounds: Common injury often stepping on an object such as a nail, common workplace injury
- **Imaging:** XR: evaluation of location or retention of FB

  MRI: Preoperative planning to rule out osteomyelitis
- **Organisms:**
  - *Staphylococcus aureus:* Most common soft tissue infection
  - *Pseudomonas:* Most common osteomyelitis
- **Treatment:**
  - **Nonoperative:** Acute injury: Bedside I&D, tetanus, abx that cover pseudomonas
  - **Operative:** Tract and soft tissue debridement removal of any devitalized bone, post-op quinolones preferred abx

Abbreviations

Abx = antibiotics
BM = bone matrix
Cx = culture
DBM = demineralized bone matrix
DM = diabetes
Dx = diagnosis
Histo = histology
HO = heterotopic ossification
LDH = lactate dehydrogenase
Osteo = osteomyelitis
RT-PCR = reverse transcriptase PCR
XR = X-ray

JILLIAN M. KAZLEY • MATTHEW R. DICAPRIO

BENIGN SOFT TISSUE TUMORS

Pigmented Villonodular Synovitis
- **Background:** Monoarticular proliferation of synovial tissue. Two types localized and diffuse (*Radiology* 2008;246:662; *Foot Ankle Spec* 2016;9:58)
  - **Localized pigmented villonodular synovitis (PVNS):** Invades one aspect of a joint and usually responds well to treatment
  - **Diffuse PVNS:** Widespread involving the entire joint, more damaging and difficult to treat
  - 5q33 chromosomal rearrangement causing ↑*CSF1* gene
- **Presentation:** Pain, swelling, limited ROM, recurrent hemarthrosis. Ankle is the third most common location.
- **Imaging/Dx:** Arthrocentesis: hemarthrosis, scope will show reddish brown synovium with papillary projections, may biopsy to confirm dx
  - **XR:** Cystic erosion and sclerotic borders of the joint
  - **MRI:** Well-circumscribed, blooming artifact—iron in hemosiderin causing signal interference
- **Histo:** Hemosiderin-stained multinucleated giant cells, pigmented foam (lipid histiocytes) cells
- **Treatment:** Synovectomy—if symptomatic, most common complication is recurrence
  CSF 1 antibody targeted treatments currently under clinical trials (*Curr Opin Oncol* 2011;23:361)

GCT Tendon Sheath (Pigmented Villonodular Tumor of the Tendon Sheath)
- **Background:** Benign nodular tumor
- **Presentation:** Firm enlarging nodular mass painless or painful with activity/ROM
- **Imaging/Dx:** XR: 5% to 15% pressure erosion of the bone
  MRI: Solid nodular mass with areas of signal void because of hemosiderin deposits
- **Histo:** Foamy histiocytes, hemosiderin, and multinucleated giant cells common
- **Treatment:** Surgical excision; recurrence is common

Plantar Fibromatosis (Ledderhose Disease)
- **Background:** Benign proliferation of myofibroblasts and collagen similar to Dupuytren contracture
- **Presentation:** Painful mass along the plantar aponeurosis on the bottom of the foot
- **Treatment:** Conservative orthotics and steroid injections often require surgical excision/plantar fasciectomy if symptomatic, unfortunately high recurrence rate up to 90%

Ganglion Cysts
- **Background:** Mucin-filled synovial cysts
- **Presentation:** Usually asymptomatic, palpable firm well-circumscribed mass, it may get irritated by shoes/clothing or just cosmetically unpleasing
- **Imaging/Dx:** XR: normal
  MRI: Not needed, but would show homogenous fluid in a well-circumscribed cavity
- **Histo:** Synovial cells with mucin accumulation
- **Treatment:** Observation, often resolves without intervention
- Aspiration/closed rupture not usually recommend and have a high rate of recurrence
  Surgical resection only if long-standing symptoms and conservative measures have failed, has much lower rate of recurrence

Hemangiomas
- **Background:** Vascular tumor
- **Presentation:** Pain, position-dependent swelling of tumors
- **Imaging/Dx:** XR: may have small phleboliths within the lesion
  MRI: A determinant lesion on MRI with characteristic "bag of worms"—heterogeneous lesion with small blood vessels and fatty infiltration
- **Histo:** Abundance of vascular dilatations and adipose
- **Treatment:** Observation, NSAIDs, compression stockings, activity modification
  Sclerotherapy/embolization failed conservative management
  Surgical excision for lesions failing conservative management, high rate of local recurrence

Schwannomas
- **Background:** Peripheral nerve sheath tumor
- **Presentation:** Usually asymptomatic, may have paresthesias, tend to occur on flexor surfaces, associated with *NF2* gene

- **Imaging/Dx:** MRI: "sting sign" signal uptake
- **Histo:** Verocay bodies: rows of cells in palisading formation
  - **Antoni A:** Organized spindle cells with staggered arrangement
  - **Antoni B:** Loosely arranged spindle cells
  - **Immunostain:** +S100 AB
- **Treatment:** Usually observation; marginal excision if symptomatic

---

BENIGN BONE TUMORS

Subungual Exostosis
- **Background:** Osteocartilaginous tumors occurring beneath the nail bed most commonly of the great toe. It is a fibrocartilaginous proliferation that undergoes endochondral ossification.
- **Presentation:** Often have pain, swelling, possible ulceration over the nail, mostly children with a hx of trauma or infection
- **Imaging/Dx:** XR: osseous and usually appear well circumscribed, no clear connection to the medullary canal or cortex unlike osteochondromas
- **Treatment:** Incision and removal of the fibrocartilaginous cap minimizes recurrence, nail bed may need to be removed (*J Bone Oncol* 2015;4:37).

Chondroblastomas
- **Background:** Aggressive tumor with high rate of recurrence
- **Presentation:** Usually teenager with mild progressive pain, limp, ↓ROM, can be found in the distal tibia, calcaneus
- **Imaging/Dx:** Well-circumscribed lytic epiphyseal lesion with sclerotic borders, may have stippled calcifications within lesion, cortical expansion
- **Histo:** Chondroblasts in "chicken wire-calcifications"/"cobblestone" appearance from plump chondroblasts, multinucleated giant cells
- **Treatment:** Rx: extended curettage and bone grafting ± adjuvant therapy if symptomatic, resection if pulmonary mets

Osteoid Osteoma/Osteoblastoma
- **Background:** Osteoid osteoma nidus <2 cm, similar histologically for osteoblastoma but with a nidus >2 cm
- **Presentation:** Dull, achy pain; osteoid osteoma pain responsive to NSAIDs, whereas osteoblastomas are not, may cause swelling or limp, may be found in tubular bones of the foot, calcaneus

- **Imaging/Dx:** XR: lytic or lytic/blastic lesion with reactive sclerotic border that expands into soft tissue and cortical thinning
- **Histo:** Abundance of giant cells, nidus has osteoblastic rimming of immature osteoid
- **Treatment:** Curettage and excision with bone grafting; radiofrequency with ablation

Enchondroma
- **Background:** Hyaline cartilage tumor caused by incomplete endochondral ossification
- **Presentation:** Asymptomatic, or may cause pain or pathologic stress fractures
- **Imaging/Dx:** XR: diaphyseal/metaphyseal, well circumscribed, may cause cortical expansion and thinning, stippling- "popcorn" appearance
  Bone scan: Can be helpful if systemic diseases like Ollier or Maffucci syndrome are suspected, but usually not indicated
  MRI: May help to assess for local extension or periosteal reaction which can help differentiate from aggressive lesions
- **Histo:** Bland hyaline cartilage encased in normal bone
- **Treatment:** Typically observation, curettage and bone grafting for impending fracture or recurrent fracture

Nonossifying Fibroma
- **Background:** Most common benign bone tumor of childhood; lesions often heal on their own after skeletal maturity
- **Presentation:** Asymptomatic usually found incidentally or after pathologic fractures
- **Imaging/Dx:** XR; eccentric metaphyseal lobular lytic lesion with well-circumscribed sclerotic borders
- **Histo:** Bland spindle cells in a whirling pattern "helicopter in a wheat field," giant cells, hemosiderin
- **Treatment:** Observation: most lesions resolve, curettage and bone grafting in symptomatic/large lesion >50% cortical diameter

Giant Cell Tumor
- **Background:** Benign but aggressive
- **Presentation:** Painful, often palpable mass, decreased ROM, possible pathologic fracture
- **Imaging/Dx:** XR: eccentric metaphyseal lesion that can extend into the epiphysis and subchondral plate lytic lesion ± cortical erosion well-circumscribed lesion, "soap bubble" appearance
  - **MRI:** Clearly defines the lesion, evaluation for soft tissue extension
  - **CXR:** For lung mets

- **Histo:** Abundance of multinucleated giant cells where the nuclei of stromal cells match the nuclei of giant cells
- **Treatment:** Operative: extended curettage with use of adjuvants; filling of void with bone graft and/or cement
  Nonoperative: Radiation only for inoperable lesions, medical management with bisphosphonate or denosumab

Aneurysmal Bone Cyst
- **Background:** Lesion with multiloculated blood-filled cavities, can be locally destructive
- **Presentation:** Pain, swelling, pathologic fracture
- **Imaging/Dx:** Eccentric lytic lobular lesion usually at the metaphysis that is expansile
- **MRI:** Multiple fluid-fluid levels, the lesion may expand into soft tissue
- **Histo:** Cavity of blood-filled spaces or "lakes of blood" surrounded by benign giant cells
- **Treatment:** Observation, extended curettage and adjuvants with bone grafting if symptomatic

Simple Bone Cyst
- **Background:** Serous-filled lesion
- **Presentation:** Asymptomatic, pathologic fracture, often young adults—may resolve after skeletal maturity
- **Imaging/Dx:** XR: central lytic lesion, thinning of cortices at metaphysis in proximity to the physis early in childhood but grows away from physis toward diaphysis during skeletal growth
  - **"Fallen leaf" sign:** Cortical fragment falling to base of cyst after pathologic fracture
  - **MRI:** Will show rim enhancement of cystic lesion
- **Histo:** Fibrous tissue, giant cells, hemosiderin pigment, uniform spindle cells
- **Treatment**
  - Majority treated with observation
  - Aspiration and injection (cortisone; BM; DBM)
  - Extended curettage and bone grafting for recalcitrant lesion

---

MALIGNANT SOFT TISSUE TUMORS

Acral Lentiginous Melanoma
- **Background**
  - ABCDEs (Asymmetry, Border irregularity, Color variation, Diameter >6 mm, Elevated/Enlarging)

- Depth is the most important prognostic factor, >4.0 mm survival ~50%
- Subungual subtype with black vertical line on the nail, poor prognosis 5 years ~50% survival
- **Presentation:** Acral lentiginous melanoma lower extremity lesions often on great toe
- **Imaging/Dx:** Biopsy of the nail bed and matrix
- **Histo:** Melanocytes with cellular atypia, invasion into the dermis, hyperchromatic nuclei with prominent nucleoli
- **Treatment:** Based on size: local excision <2 mm thick, may need sentinel node biopsy if >1 mm thick, complete local excision with wide margins/amputations

Synovial Sarcoma
- **Background:** Most common malignant sarcoma of the foot, t (X:18) chromosomal translocation creating fusion gene *SYT-SSX*, metastasize often to the lung and lymph nodes
- **Presentation:** Young adults, often painful, palpable mass $\pm$ lymphadenopathy
- **Imaging/Dx:** 30% soft tissue calcification and mimic appearance of HO
- **Histo:** Monophasic—mostly spindle cells or biphasic-spindle cells and epithelial cells
- **Treatment:** Wide surgical resection with consideration of adjuvant chemo and radiation for tumors >5 cm

---

MALIGNANT BONE TUMORS

Chondrosarcoma
- **Background:** Cartilaginous tumor
  - Telomerase activity can be determined by RT-PCR and is directly related to recurrence.
  - Most commonly met to lung
- **Presentation:** Pain or mass; occasionally pathologic fracture
- **Imaging/Dx:** XR: endosteal erosion/scalloping, cortical thickening, ill-defined margins, matrix calcification, may have soft tissue extension
  - **MRI:** Heterogeneous, multilobulated appearance is helpful in making the diagnosis; look for soft tissue component
  - Similar appearance to enchondroma get MRI if concern/lesions >5 cm
- **Histo:** chondrocytes $\pm$ atypia; cartilage invading bone; loss of encasement pattern
- **Treatment:** Wide surgical excision, amputation

Osteosarcoma
- **Background:** *Rb* gene, elevated alk phos
- **Presentation:** Pain, swelling, most commonly present at stage 2B
- **Imaging/Dx:** XR: blastic and destructive, Codman triangle-periosteal reaction, Sun burst—periosteal elevation
  - **MRI:** Eval soft tissue involvement or skip mets
  - **CT chest:** Look for pulmonary mets
  - **Biopsy:** Should be done by surgeon providing definite care
- **Histo:** Malignant spindle cells producing osteoid
- **Treatment:** Multiagent chemo, wide surgical resection (limb salvage vs amputation)

Ewing Sarcoma
- **Background:** Young adults first two decades of life, translocation 11:22 creating the *EWS-FLI1* gene, may have a *p53* mutation
- **Presentation:** Pain, swelling ± fever
- **Imaging/Dx:** Lytic diaphysis or metaphysis lesion with "moth eaten" appearance, periosteal reaction can show "onion skinning"
  - **Workup:** ↑ESR, ↑WBC, ↓H/H, ↑LDH, bone marrow biopsy
  - **Bone scan:** Help staging, hot lesions
  - **MRI:** Eval soft tissue involvement—often extensive, help staging
- **Histo:** Small round blue cells
- **Treatment:** Multiagent neoadjuvant and maintenance chemo with wide surgical resection/amputation
  Radiation if positive surgical margins or surgical resection too morbid (spine; certain pelvic tumors)

Metastatic Lesions
- Uncommon in foot and ankle
- Renal and lung carcinomas are the two most common primary carcinomas to be found distal to the knee.

JILLIAN M. KAZLEY • MATTHEW R. DICAPRIO

SOFT TISSUE RECONSTRUCTION

Considerations: The foot and ankle region presents unique issues when it comes to soft tissue reconstruction.
- Must consider size, location, weight bearing versus non–weight bearing
  - Weight-bearing surfaces: It is ideal to have sensation in the coverage area to prevent ulcerations/breakdown.
  - Limited tissue mobility based on multiple areas of adherence (*Front Surg* 2016;3:15)

Coverage Option	Uses	Advantages	Disadvantages
Local advancement	Wound $< 3\ cm^2$	Avoids surplus tissue	Only small wounds
Skin grafting	Wound $> 3\ cm^2$ Dorsum of the foot, NWB instep	Simple procedure	Insensate, needs well-vascularized wound bed, DM/ smoking may compromise graft
Flaps	Wound $> 3\ cm^2$ Plantar WB areas	Durable	May provide surplus tissue, can be thinned out over time

Flaps
- **Sural flap:** Local flap, small defects of the hindfoot over the malleoli, only good for small defects due to limited arterial supply from sural artery, insensate
- **Anterior lateral thigh flap:** Free flap, versatile and can cover larger defects, sensation from lateral femoral cutaneous
- Instep—island flap—local flap using medial plantar artery and nerve, small defects of the WB hindfoot, sensation from medial plantar

MIDFOOT ARTHRITIS

JASON P. TARTAGLIONE • MAXWELL C. ALLEY • JORDAN M. LISELLA •
ANTHONY P. MECHREFE • ROBERT L. PARISIEN

MIDFOOT ANATOMY

- Spans from transverse tarsal joint to the tarsometatarsal joints
- Archlike bony anatomy as well as recessed 2nd metatarsal (MT) provide inherent bony stability to the midfoot
- **Bones:** Navicular, medial/middle/lateral cuneiforms, cuboid
- Joints
  - TMT (tarsometatarsal/Lisfranc joint)
  - NC (naviculocuneiform)
  - TN (talonavicular)
  - CC (calcaneocuboid)
    - Columns
      - **Medial:** 1st ray; medial cuneiform and 1st MT
      - **Middle:** 2nd and 3rd ray; intermediate and lateral cuneiforms and 2nd and 3rd MT
      - **Lateral:** 4th and 5th ray; cuboid and 4th and 5th MT
- Ligaments
  - Strong ligamentous structures stabilize the TMT joints
  - **Lisfranc ligament:** Interosseous ligament spanning from the medial cuneiform to the 2nd MT
  - Ligamentous anatomy divided into plantar, interosseous, and dorsal structures (interosseous and plantar ligaments are stronger than dorsal, therefore bony displacement after injury is commonly dorsal)
  - **Intermetatarsal ligaments:** Span between the bases of the 2nd to 5th MT, absent ligamentous attachment between 1st and 2nd MT

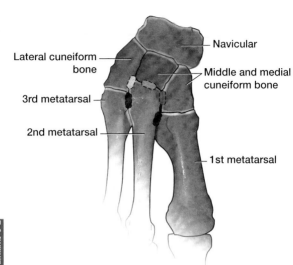

1st-3rd ray anatomy demonstrating the recessed 2nd MT within the midfoot.

From Easley ME, Wiesel SW. Operative Techniques in Foot and Ankle Surgery. 2nd ed. Philadelphia, PA: Wolters Kluwer; 2017.

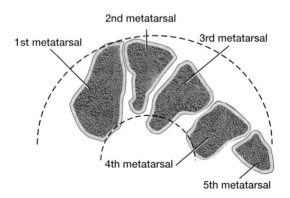

Axial image demonstrating the arch like anatomy of the midfoot.

From Easley ME, Wiesel SW. Operative Techniques in Foot and Ankle Surgery. 2nd ed. Philadelphia, PA: Wolters Kluwer; 2017.

MIDFOOT BIOMECHANICS

- Allows transmittance of load from the hindfoot to the forefoot, serves as lever arm
- Very little motion
- Acts as a roman arch in the axial plane, with the base of the 2nd MT acting as the keystone
- Variable dorsiflexion and mechanical coupling of the forefoot to the hindfoot depending on gait
- Lateral column significantly more mobile than medial or middle column

ETIOLOGY

- Posttraumatic-primary cause
  - Most common midfoot injury is to the Lisfranc joint complex
    - Outcomes correlate with degree of anatomic incongruency
  - Injuries to navicular and cuboid can also lead to significant arthrosis of the TMT joint complex
- Other etiologies include DJD/OA, inflammatory arthritis, crystalline arthropathy, neuropathic degeneration, and structural abnormalities secondary to advanced adult acquired flat foot deformity

CLINICAL MANIFESTATIONS

- Presents with pain at the affected joint(s)
- Midfoot collapse may or may not be present
- **Age:** Bimodal distribution—posttraumatic etiology in younger patients and degenerative causes in older patients
- TMT arthritis may present with deformity including pes planovalgus, hallux valgus, or rocker-bottom deformity
- Osteophytes may be palpable on the dorsum of the foot, which may be painful in certain footwear
- **Piano key test:** Plantarly directed force applied to the metatarsal head elicits pain in the respective TMT joint

RADIOGRAPHIC EXAMINATION

- Workup should include weight-bearing AP, lateral, and internal rotation oblique foot radiographs
  - On the lateral, sagging of the medial column at either the TMT or the NC joint indicates midfoot instability and collapse
  - On the AP, TMT diastasis can be appreciated
- On all images, joint space narrowing, subluxation, and osteophyte formation can be noted

NONOPERATIVE MANAGEMENT

- First-line treatment
- In general, focus on improving midfoot stability and offloading arthritic joints
- Activity modification
- **NSAIDs:** First-line treatment of any arthritic joint pain, though extended use is undesirable due to side effects
- Shoe modifications and orthotic inserts
  - **Benefits:** Designed to facilitate the transfer of weight during gait
  - **Drawbacks:** May be viewed as cumbersome, temporary
  - **Examples:** Orthotics, stiff soled shoes, and rocker bottom shoes
  - Polypropylene ankle-foot clamshell orthosis can offload the plantar foot by as much as 30% (*Foot Ankle* 1992;13:14)

OPERATIVE MANAGEMENT

- **Indications:** Failure of nonoperative management
- **Contraindications:** Active infection, uncontrolled medical comorbidities, ischemic/neuropathic foot, active smoker (relative)
- **Medial and middle column:** Arthrodesis of medial and middle columns is gold standard
  - **Pre-op:** Identify problematic joints w/clinical and radiographic examination, $\pm$ image guided anesthetic injection of suspected joints
  - Outcomes
    - Significant improvements in pain, gait, and alignment noted on AOFAS scores and improvements in pain, disability, and activity limitations
    - Quality of anatomic reduction is most important predictor of outcome in cases of posttraumatic arthritis
- **Lateral column:** More debate
  - **Lateral column arthrodesis:** Less support than medial and middle column arthrodesis
    - Lateral column is more mobile relative to medial and middle columns
    - Increased rate of complications including nonunion, chronic lateral foot pain, stress fractures, prominent/broken hardware
    - Good outcomes observed in cases of lateral midfoot collapse, rocker-bottom deformity, and Charcot arthropathy
- **Motion preserving procedure:**
  - Joint debridement
  - Lateral TMT joint resection with interposition arthroplasty
    - Joints are resected, soft tissue is placed in the void
    - Lateral column motion preserved
    - 35% reduction in pain, 6/8 patients satisfied (*Foot Ankle Int* 2002;23:440)
- Surgical complications of arthrodesis
  - **Nonunion:** 3% to 7% (*Foot Ankle Int* 2007;28:482; *J Bone Joint Surg Am* 2006;88:514)
  - **Wound complications:** 3% to 5% nondiabetic; up to 53% in diabetics (*Clin Orthop Relat Res* 2001;391:45)
  - **Post-op neuroma:** 7% (*J Bone Joint Surg Am* 1996;78:1376)
  - **Symptomatic hardware:** 9%
  - **Long term:** Metatarsal stress fractures, metatarsalgia, adjacent joint arthritis, sesamoid pain

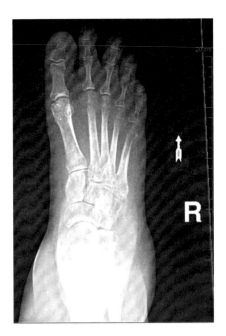

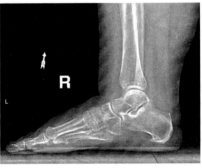

From Easley ME, Wiesel SW. *Operative Techniques in Foot and Ankle Surgery.* 2nd ed. Philadelphia, PA: Wolters Kluwer; 2017.

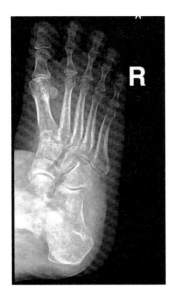

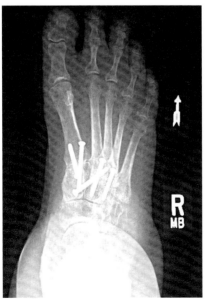

From Easley ME, Wiesel SW. *Operative Techniques in Foot and Ankle Surgery.* 2nd ed. Philadelphia, PA: Wolters Kluwer; 2017.

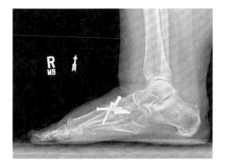

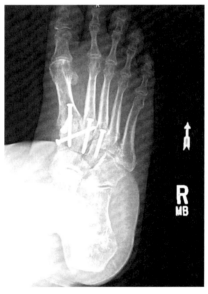

AP, lateral, and oblique radiographs demonstrating midfoot arthritis pre- and postoperatively status post midfoot fusion. (From Easley ME, Wiesel SW. *Operative Techniques in Foot and Ankle Surgery.* 2nd ed. Philadelphia, PA: Wolters Kluwer; 2017.)

HINDFOOT ARTHRITIS

JASON P. TARTAGLIONE • MAXWELL C. ALLEY • JORDAN M. LISELLA •
ANTHONY P. MECHREFE • ROBERT L. PARISIEN

HINDFOOT ANATOMY

- Hindfoot articulations include the subtalar (ST), talonavicular (TN), and calcaneocuboid (CC) joints
- Talus
  - 60% covered by articular cartilage
  - Comprised of the body, neck, head, lateral process, posterior processes (medial and lateral)
  - Articulates with the tibia, navicular, and calcaneus
  - No muscular attachments
  - Tenuous blood supply
    - Anastomotic sling created from branches off of the perforating peroneal, dorsalis pedis, and posterior tibial arteries
    - Neck fractures associated with highest risk of AVN due to retrograde blood supply
- Calcaneus
  - Comprised of the tuberosity, sustentaculum tali, and anterior process
  - Articulates with the talus, cuboid
  - Superiorly, anterior, middle, and posterior facets articular with talus
  - Strong ligamentous attachments to the talus, cuboid, and navicular
    - **Lateral:** Calcaneofibular ligament, interosseous ligament, bifurcate ligament, cervical ligament, inferior extensor retinaculum
    - **Medial:** Calcaneonavicular ligament or spring ligament
- **ST joint:** Articulation between talus and calcaneus
  - Comprised of three facets (anterior, middle, and posterior)
  - Posterior facet is saddle shaped
  - Primarily responsible for hindfoot eversion and inversion
  - Works in concert with TN and CC joints to accommodate uneven ground
- **Transverse tarsal joint (Chopart):** Consists of the CC and TN joints

HINDFOOT BIOMECHANICS

- Transverse tarsal motion is the key to the dichotomous actions of accommodating uneven ground during heel strike and allowing for rigid push off during toe off
- During heel strike, the hindfoot is in valgus, which creates parallelism between the CC and TN joints effectively unlocking the two joints and allowing motion
- During toe off, the hindfoot assumes a varus position, which creates unparallelism between the CC and TN joints effectively locking the two joints and inhibiting motion

ETIOLOGY

- Most commonly posttraumatic (calcaneus and/or talus fractures)
- Inflammatory arthritides
- Primary degenerative arthritis
- End-stage posterior tibialis tendon disorders
- Tarsal coalition
- Neuropathic arthropathies
- Following ankle fusion

CLINICAL MANIFESTATIONS AND EVALUATION

- Full comprehensive medical history
- History of trauma
- Patients complain of pain in the sinus tarsi and difficulty walking on uneven surfaces
- Pain is reproduced with hindfoot inversion and eversion
- Decreased hindfoot ROM compared to contralateral side
- The Coleman block test used to determine the hindfoot's flexibility
- Examine the patient while weight bearing to examine overall alignment

RADIOGRAPHIC EXAMINATION

- Weight-bearing AP, mortise, and lateral views of the ankle as well as weight-bearing AP, oblique, and lateral views of the foot should be obtained
- Special views
  - **Broden view:** Allows visualization of ST joint
  - **Saltzman and Harris heel views:** Used to assess varus/valgus hindfoot alignment
- A CT scan may be obtained to better elucidate the extent of hindfoot arthritis

NONOPERATIVE MANAGEMENT

- NSAIDs
- Activity modification
  - Avoid uneven terrain
  - Limit high-impact activities
- Orthoses that control hindfoot motion (ie, AFO)
  - Flexible deformities can be managed with posts and orthotics
  - Rigid deformities may be accommodated using soft, moldable materials to accommodate the deformity
- Corticosteroid injections including fluoroscopically guided injections in order to ensure proper placement
  - Has the potential to work both therapeutically and diagnostically

OPERATIVE MANAGEMENT

- Debridement (open vs arthroscopic)
- Arthrodesis
  - Selective fusion of a single hindfoot joint can be utilized for isolated arthritis with the goal of maintaining motion and limiting adjacent joint arthritis
    - **Isolated CC:** Limits hindfoot motion by about 25%
    - **Isolated ST:** Limits hindfoot motion by about 40%
    - **Isolated TN:** Limits hindfoot motion by about 90%
  - Triple arthrodesis, which encompasses the ST, TN, and CC joints, is the treatment of choice for rigid hindfoot pathology (ie, Stage 3 PTTD)
  - Various fixation techniques used to achieve fusion including headed and headless screws, plates and screws, as well as staples
  - Subtalar bone block arthrodesis is used to restore hindfoot alignment and height in the presence of loss of heel height
  - Ideal hindfoot fusion position:
    - 5 degrees of hindfoot valgus with neutral Meary angles on AP and lateral radiographs
  - **Union rates:** Isolated ST is 84% to 100% (*Foot Ankle Clin* 2011;16:83), isolated TN is 90% to 97% (*Foot Ankle Int* 2009;30:150), CC joint is rarely fused in isolation and most commonly performed in a double or triple arthrodesis
  - Triple arthrodesis (*Foot Ankle Surg* 2012:175)
    - Fusion of ST, TN, and CC joints
    - Fusion rates as high as 95%

- Allows significant correction of hindfoot malalignment
- Risk of adjacent joint degeneration
  - Ankle, 40% to 100%
  - Midfoot, 50%

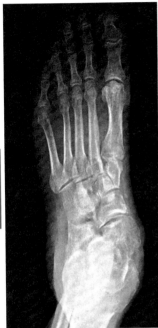

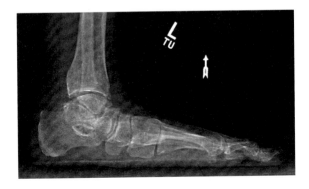

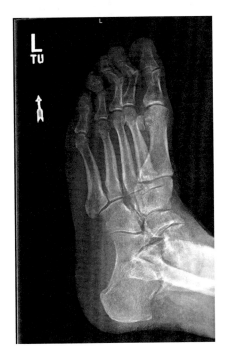

(continued)

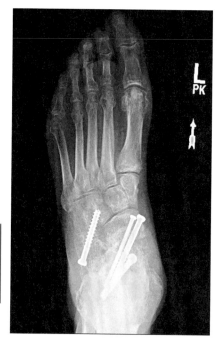

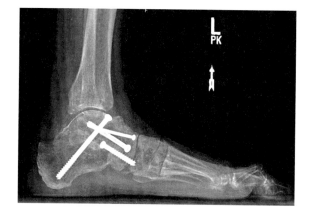

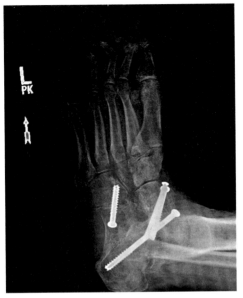

AP, lateral, and oblique images of a left foot demonstrating Stage IIIb PTTD pre- and postoperatively status post triple arthrodesis

- **Double arthrodesis:**
  - Selective fusion of two of the three hindfoot joints
  - Goal of fusing the arthritic joints and preserving motion in the nonarthritic joint in order to decrease risk of adjacent degeneration
  - Smaller incisions
  - Shorter surgery
  - less bone prep
  - less blood loss
  - one less fusion site that has to heal
- Complications
  - Wound complications
  - Prominent hardware requiring removal
  - Infection
  - Neurovascular injury
    - Highest with CC fusion, sural nerve
  - Nonunion
  - Malunion
  - Adjacent joint degeneration

JASON P. TARTAGLIONE • MAXWELL C. ALLEY • JORDAN M. LISELLA • ANTHONY P. MECHREFE • ROBERT L. PARISIEN

ANKLE ANATOMY

- The tibia and fibula create a highly constrained mortise that contains the talar dome
- Stability is provided by osseous anatomy and ligamentous complexes that provide stability in all planes and axes of motion
- The talar dome and tibial plafond are highly conforming surfaces, which enable maximal contact area and decreased contact pressure
- **Ligaments:**
  - **Lateral:** Anterior talofibular ligament (ATFL), posterior talofibular ligament (PTFL), calcaneofibular ligament (CFL)
  - **Medial:** Deltoid complex (superficial: tibionavicular, tibiocalcaneal, tibiotalar ligaments and deep deltoid ligament which is the strongest and thickest medial sided ligament)
  - **Syndesmotic ligaments:** Anterior inferior tibiofibular ligament (AITFL), posterior inferior tibiofibular ligament (PITFL), interosseous membrane (IOM), interosseous ligament (IOL), transverse ligament (posterior complex is the strongest)

PRINCIPAL GROUPS OF ANKLE LIGAMENTS

Medial Collateral (Deltoid) Ligament

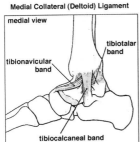

medial view

tibiotalar band

tibionavicular band

tibiocalcaneal band

Lateral Collateral Ligament

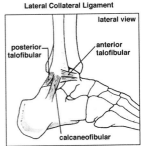

lateral view

posterior talofibular

anterior talofibular

calcaneofibular

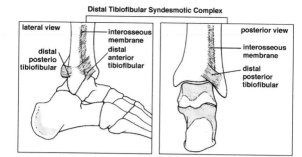

Ligaments of the ankle. Three principal sets of ligaments form the ankle joint: the medial collateral (deltoid) ligament, the lateral collateral ligament, and the distal tibiofibular syndesmotic complex, which is important for maintaining ankle integrity and stability. Greenspan A. *Orthopedic Imaging: A Practical Approach*. Philadelphia, PA: Wolters Kluwer Health/Lippincott Williams & Wilkins; 2011.

ANKLE BIOMECHANICS

- The ankle is primarily a ginglymus (hinge) joint
- Primarily plantarflexes and dorsiflexes (50°/20°) about an axis that lies between the tip of the medial and lateral malleoli with the talar dome acting as a fulcrum of a cone with its apex oriented medially
- Works in concert with the hindfoot joints to position the foot on uneven terrain
- In the normal ankle, the anatomic and mechanical axis pass through the center of the ankle joint in the coronal and sagittal planes
- Normal motion of the ankle requires the fibula to translate, rotate, and migrate with respect to the tibia
- An intact syndesmosis is crucial to maintaining normal tibiotalar as well as tibiofibular motion
  - 1 mm of lateral talar displacement in the ankle mortise generates a 42% decrease in available joint contact area resulting in an increase in contact pressure (*J Orthop Res* 2005;23:743)
- The tibiotalar joint is able to withstand 5.5 times body weight (*Clin Orthop Relat Res* 1977;127:189)
- The ankle bears the highest load per surface area of any joint in the body
- Ankle cartilage is thinner than hip or knee cartilage and is biomechanically and metabolically different from hip and knee cartilage making it more resistant to degenerative

changes (*Arthritis Rheum* 1997;26:667; *Clin Orthop Relat Res* 2009;467:1800; *Foot Ankle Clin* 2008;13:341)
- Arthritis of the ankle significantly alters gait mechanics secondary to the distal translation of the ankle joint's center of rotation

ETIOLOGY

- Ankle arthritis is a progressive condition resulting in dysfunction of hyaline cartilage, subchondral bone, and synovium
- Generally affects younger, more active, and higher demand patients
- Affects about 1% of the population (*Clin Orthop Relat Res* 2009;467:1800)
- Unlike the hip and knee, ankle arthritis is most commonly posttraumatic in nature
  - Pilon injuries, ankle fractures/dislocations, talus fractures
  - Radiographic changes usually apparent by 2 years after injury although pain may be delayed for years
  - Severity of arthritis is related to initial injury pattern as well as articular congruency
- Other causes
  - Inflammatory diseases
  - Chronic ligamentous instability
  - AVN
  - Septic arthritis
  - Peripheral neuropathy
  - Degenerative osteoarthritis
- Estimated annual cost of LE posttraumatic arthritis is $12 billion in the United States (*J Orthop Trauma* 2006;20:749)
- Has been shown to be as disabling as knee and hip OA (*J Bone Joint Surg Am* 2008;90:499)

CLINICAL MANIFESTATIONS AND EVALUATION

- Comprehensive history and physical
- Antalgic gait with decreased walking speed, cadence, and stride length
- Pain over anterior ankle (worse with range of motion [ROM], weight bearing, and during push-off)
- Joint effusion may be palpable
- Decreased ROM
- Increased pressure experienced by adjacent hindfoot joints
- Alignment should be evaluated with the patient standing

- No current labs are helpful in making the dx of arthritis; however, if there is concern for infectious etiology, WBC, ESR, and CRP should be reviewed

RADIOGRAPHIC EXAMINATION

- Weight-bearing AP, mortise, and lateral views of the ankle
  - Assess joint space narrowing, alignment, subchondral cysts, osteophytes, AVN
- In addition, AP, lateral, and oblique weight-bearing images of the foot should be reviewed to assess for deformity and concomitant pathology

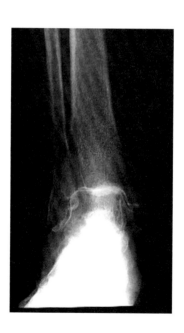

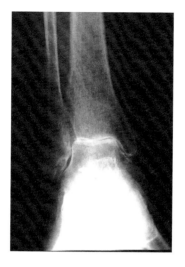

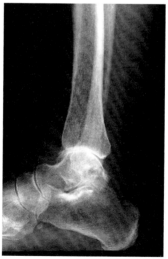

AP, mortise, and lateral images of a right ankle demonstrating ankle arthritis

NONOPERATIVE MANAGEMENT

- First-line treatment modality
- Goal is to relieve symptoms and prolong the life and function of the native ankle
- Effectiveness related to severity of arthritis
- NSAIDs
- Activity modification (low impact exercises and activities like swimming or stationary bike)
- Weight loss
- Assistive devices
- Corticosteroid injections (can be both diagnostic and therapeutic)
- Viscosupplementation has been used but there is little literature to support its use in the ankle
- Bracing (ie, AFO) or short-term immobilization (ie, CAM walker boot) limiting tibiotalar motion and decreasing pain

OPERATIVE MANAGEMENT

- Indicated when nonoperative measures fail to improve pain/dysfunction and the patient is medically appropriate for surgery
- Severity of symptoms, level of activity, occupation, patient age, and comorbidities are all used to help determine whether to use joint-sparing or joint-sacrificing techniques

JOINT SPARING

- Arthroscopic versus open debridement for milder stages of arthritis
  - Exostectomy
  - Debridement of hypertrophic synovium
  - Removal of loose bodies
  - Drilling of osteochondral lesions
  - Cartilage rejuvenation procedures
  - Osteochondral allograft transplantation (OATS)
  - Chondrocyte transplantation
- Supramalleolar osteotomy
  - When symptoms are secondary to tibiotalar malalignment
  - Indicated for mild disease with eccentric articular wear patterns and relatively preserved ROM
- Distraction arthroplasty
  - Alternative to ankle fusion and ankle arthroplasty

- Uses external fixator, usually with a hinge to allow ROM, to mechanically unload the articular cartilage through joint distraction
- Exact mechanism unknown; however, the theory is to allow cartilage regeneration in the setting of an unloaded joint surface and a well-aligned limb
- Consider in younger patients who are motivated and compliant
- Patients generally allowed to bear weight
- Goals are to maintain motion, relieve pain, delay or prevent progression of arthritis
- High patient burden
- Less common than fusion or arthroplasty; however, recent studies demonstrate that distraction arthroplasty is a reasonable option in the appropriately selected patient (*Foot Ankle Int* 2009;30:318; *J Orthop Res* 2014;32:96)

JOINT SACRIFICING

- Arthrodesis
  - Ankle fusion is considered the "gold standard"
  - Provides predictable pain relief
  - However, the loss of ankle motion alters gait kinematics leading to increased stress on adjacent joints with progressive degeneration and increased energy expenditure
  - Can be performed arthroscopically, through a mini-arthrotomy, or using open techniques with internal and/or external fixation
- **Optimal fusion position:** Neutral plantarflexion/dorsiflexion and 5 degrees of valgus with rotation equal to contralateral leg or 5 degrees of external rotation
- **Disadvantages:**
  - Prolonged postoperative immobilization
  - Progression of arthritis in adjacent hindfoot joints (reported as high as 90%) (*J Bone Joint Surg Am* 2001;83-A:219)
  - Gait abnormalities
  - Negatively affects functional status
    - Difficulty putting on shoes/boots
    - Difficulty rising from a chair
    - Altering use of driving pedals
    - Difficulty ascending and descending stairs

- Difficulty walking on uneven ground
- Difficulty kneeling
- Alters the fashion in which objects are picked up off of the floor
- Decreased physical and emotional subscores on SF-36 testing
- Risk of delayed union, nonunion (ranges from 7% to 43%) (*Foot Ankle Int* 1994;15:581; *Foot Ankle Int* 2013;34:557), and symptomatic pseudoarthrosis (higher in smokers)
- Infection
  - Wound breakdown
  - Superficial and deep infections
  - Higher rates in smokers, DM, and patients with renal disease

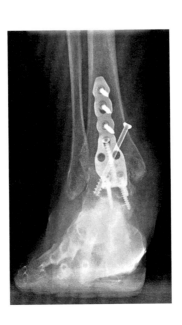

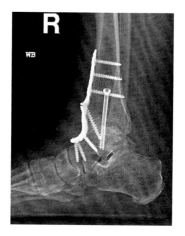

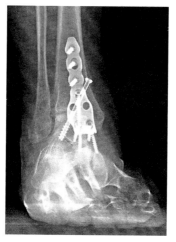

AP, lateral, and mortise radiographs of a right ankle demonstrating an ankle arthrodesis

- Arthroplasty
  - First total ankle replacement (TAR) performed in 1970
  - Since that time, new surgical techniques, improved instrumentation, and clinical experience have expanded the indications for TAR
  - Modern TAR designs and techniques have demonstrated equivalent pain relief and better function when compared with arthrodesis (*Foot Ankle Int* 2009;30:579; *J Bone Joint Surg Am* 2007;89:1899)
  - Modern TAR can replicate near-normal ankle kinematics, which is believed to decrease the mobility and stress experienced by joints distal to the ankle ultimately delaying the progression of arthritis in the adjacent hindfoot joints
  - Studies have demonstrated improvements in pain, function, quality of life, patient-reported outcomes, temporospatial parameters, and kinematic and kinetic function following TAR (*Foot Ankle Int* 2004;25:377; *Foot Ankle Int* 2008;29:3; *Foot Ankle Int* 2015;36:11; *Foot Ankle Int* 2015;36:143; *Foot Ankle Int* 2015;36:518; *Foot Ankle Int* 2016;37:938; *J Bone Joint Surg Am* 2014;96:1983)
  - Deformity should be corrected at the time of replacement or as a staged procedure in order to better recreate normal tibiotalar biomechanics
  - The recent increase in TAR demonstrates the generalized excitement both from physicians and patients alike
  - **Disadvantages:**
    - Critics cite high early failure rates
      - Wound problems
      - Infection (superficial and deep)
      - Component subsidence
      - Osteolysis
      - Malleolar fractures
      - Aseptic and septic component loosening
      - High rates of secondary procedures
        - The most common is guttural debridement
    - However, long-term implant survival is possible with surgeon experience, better designs and techniques, and appropriate indications and patient expectations
    - Long-term data with the current TAR systems are needed to better elucidate long-term outcomes

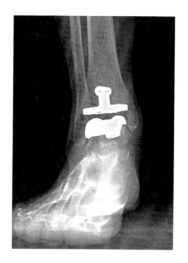

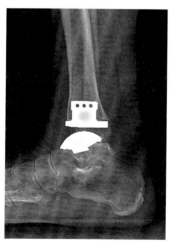

(continued)

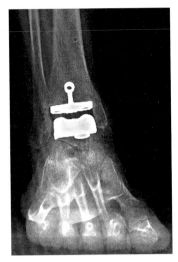

AP, lateral, and mortise radiographs of a right ankle demonstrating a total ankle replacement

From Easley ME, Wiesel SW. *Operative Techniques in Foot and Ankle Surgery*. Philadelphia, PA: Wolters Kluwer; 2017.

AAFD

MOSTAFA M. ABOUSAYED • CHRISTOPHER K. JOHNSON •
JOHN A. DIPRETA • ROBERT L. PARISIEN

A complex deformity representing collapse of the medial
longitudinal arch

ETIOLOGY

- Posterior tibial tendon dysfunction (PTTD) is the most
  common etiology; others include neuromuscular, traumatic,
  and arthritic conditions (*Foot Ankle Clin* 2007;12:233; *Foot
  Ankle Clin* 2007;12:341).

ANATOMY AND PATHOPHYSIOLOGY

- Posterior tibial muscle runs behind the axis of the ankle
  joint (ankle plantar flexor) and medial to the subtalar joint
  (hindfoot invertor).
- Other structures involved include the spring, interosseous
  talocalcaneal and deltoid ligaments.
- PTTD → collapse of the medial arch → (1) hindfoot valgus,
  (2) abduction of midfoot at transverse tarsal joint → talar
  head uncoverage, (3) compensatory forefoot supination and
  (4) Achilles contracture with subsequent equinus deformity

CLINICAL PICTURE

- Thorough history and physical examination are key to
  diagnosis.
- Pain usually starts at the medial side of the ankle, ++
  (increases) with prolonged standing.
- At later stages, patients experience lateral-sided pain
  with severe hindfoot valgus → sinus tarsi or subfibular
  impingement.
- On examination, there is tenderness along the PTT ±
  swelling. Hindfoot valgus and midfoot abduction (too many
  toes sign) become obvious as the deformity progresses.
- Posterior tibial tendon edema has 88% sensitivity and 100%
  specificity in diagnosing posterior tibial tendon pathology
  (*Foot Ankle Int* 2011;32(2):189).
- Single- and double-heel rise test are valuable in diagnosing
  PTTD (**Fig. 7-1**).

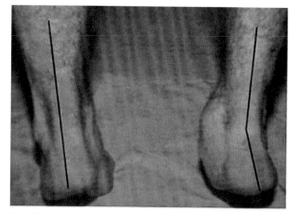

Figure 7-1 Heel rise test showing normal hindfoot alignment on the left side and valgus alignment of AAFD on the right side.

IMAGING

- Weight-bearing plain X-rays of the foot and ankle are usually adequate for diagnosis and planning management.
- Several parameters can be assessed in the AP and lateral radiographs.
- Meary's angle (lateral talus-1st metatarsal angle) helps localize the site of the sag of the medial arch (**Fig. 7-2**).
- The Saltzman (hindfoot alignment) view has gained popularity and became part of the standard radiographs.

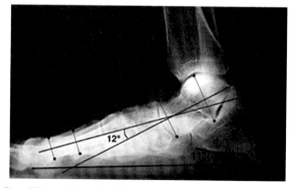

Figure 7-2 Lateral plain radiograph demonstrating lateral talus-1st metatarsal angle of 12° (normal 0°±4°) and calcaneal pitch angle (normal 17°-30°) or decreased before calcaneal pitch angle to be consistent with the lateral radiograph shown in cavus chapter.

- MRI is not routinely obtained, but can help assess the condition of the PTT and spring ligament preoperatively and aid in surgical planning.
- Other modalities have been described and can be useful, including ultrasonography, tendoscopy, and multiplanar weight-bearing images.

STAGES

- Johnson and Strom devised their classification system in 1989. Based on anatomic, pathologic, and clinical findings, it remains the most commonly used and cited classification system (*Clin Orthop* 1989;239:196).
- Myerson et al. proposed a stage IV modification of the original classification, which included advanced stages with ankle involvement (*Instr Course Lect* 1997;46:393).

Stage	Pathology	Clinical Picture	Imaging
Stage I	Normal tendon length	• Mild pain medially • Tenderness and swelling along PTT • No deformity appreciated • Able to do heel rise test	No deformity
Stage II	Elongated tendon with longitudinal tears	• Moderate pain • Flexible deformity • Weakness on heel rise test • Too-many-toes sign	**IIA:** <30% talar head uncoverage **IIB:** >30% talar head uncoverage
Stage III	Visible tears or complete rupture of the tendon	• Severe pain • ±Lateral-sided pain • Fixed deformity • Severe weakness on heel rise test or unable to do the test	Arthritis of the subtalar and transverse tarsal joints
Stage IV		• Ankle pain • Valgus ankle deformity	**IVA:** Lateral talar tilt with flexible deformity and without ankle arthritis **IVB:** Ankle arthritis with fixed ankle deformity

Conservative Treatment
- Is the first line of management of all stages
- Is highly successful in stage I (up to 90% success rate)
- It includes immobilization in a brace in the acute inflammatory phase (Arizona brace, AFO, DUAFO).
- NSAIDs can be helpful and physical therapy can be initiated after acute phase subsides (*Foot Ankle Int* 2006;27(1):2; *Foot Ankle Int* 1996;17(12):736).

Surgical Treatment
- Indicated after failure of conservative treatment
- Patient factors (eg, diabetes, smoking, and PVD should be taken into consideration)

Stage I
- Tenosynovectomy, PTT debridement, and FDL transfer have been described, though rarely indicated.

Stage II
- Controversy still exists regarding the best surgical modality.
- Several options have been described in the literature with variable success rates.
- Good results have been reported with medializing calcaneal osteotomy (MCO), FDL transfer, and lateral column lengthening (LCL) (*HSS J* 2006;2(2):157).

Stage	Operative Treatment
Stage I (rarely indicated)	• Tenosynovectomy • PTT debridement • FDL transfer
Stage II	• FDL transfer, MCO, and LCL • Cotton osteotomy vs 1st TMT fusion • Subtalar arthroereisis • Spring ligament reconstruction
Stage III	• Triple arthrodesis • Double arthrodesis (CC joint spared)
Stage IV	• Flatfoot reconstruction + deltoid ligament repair (stage IVA) • Flatfoot reconstruction + TAR vs ankle fusion (stage IVB)

AAFD 7-4

- Forefoot supination is addressed with Cotton (medial cuneiform dorsal opening wedge) osteotomy or 1st TMT fusion in the presence of medial column instability or arthritis.
- Several techniques have been described for LCL; however, regardless of the technique, they are associated with morbidities (+lateral plantar pressures, excessive stiffness, and 5th metatarsal fractures) (*Foot Ankle* 1993;14(3):136; *J Bone Joint Surg Am* 2010;92(1):81).
- Spring ligament reconstruction has recently become a popular strategy particularly in stage IIB with +++ midfoot abduction.
- Subtalar arthroereisis has been associated with good midterm results and can be useful in certain cases.

Stage III
- Triple arthrodesis is the gold standard treatment.
- In limited cases, the calcaneocuboid joint can be spared (theoretically preserving motion at the mobile column of the foot).

Stage IV
- Flatfoot reconstruction with deltoid ligament reconstruction can be done in flexible deformity without ankle arthritis.
- In stage IVB, flatfoot reconstruction with TAR versus ankle fusion is usually indicated.

CONCLUSION

- AAFD remains to be a challenging problem to orthopedic surgeons.
- No consensus exists regarding treatment, particularly stage II.
- Every attempt should be made to preserve motion.
- Arthrodesis is associated with poor outcomes, hence the trend toward earlier surgical management and deformity correction before arthritis occurs.

PES CAVUS

MOSTAFA M. ABOUSAYED • CHRISTOPHER K. JOHNSON •
JOHN A. DIPRETA • ROBERT L. PARISIEN

A spectrum of deformities characterized mainly by accentuated medial longitudinal arch. The majority of cases encompass hindfoot varus, plantarflexed 1st ray, and forefoot adduction. The primary deformity can be in the forefoot, hindfoot, or a combination of both.

ETIOLOGY

Pathophysiology
- Muscular imbalance is present in all cases regardless of the etiology.
- The combination of weak tibialis anterior and peroneus brevis and relatively stronger tibialis posterior and peroneus longus → plantarflexed 1st ray and hindfoot varus
- Recruitment of extrinsic extensors:
  - EHL → ++1st ray hyperflexion via windlass mechanism of plantar fascia
  - EDL (in combination with intrinsic weakness) → claw toes
- Equinus contracture develops (Achilles unopposed by the weak tibialis anterior)
- Contracture of plantar fascia → ++forefoot adduction and hindfoot varus
- Hindfoot locked in varus→−−transverse tarsal joint motion→−−ability of foot to adjust to uneven surface and −−ability of foot to absorb impact → overloaded 1st metatarsal head and lateral border of the foot (*Clin Orthop* 1989;246:273; *Foot Ankle Int* 1995;16:624)
- Relative talus dorsiflexion → limited ankle dorsiflexion, anterior ankle impingement. In combination with varus hindfoot → ++ contact at the anteromedial ankle → lateral talar tilt → lateral ankle instability and ankle arthritis (*Foot Ankle Int* 2002;23:1031; *Am J Sports Med* 2006;34:612)
- Deformities are flexible initially and become fixed over time.

Neuromuscular	• Hereditary motor and sensory neuropathies (eg, Charcot-Marie-Tooth [CMT]) • Cerebral palsy • Spinal tumors • Friedreich ataxia • Muscular dystrophies
Congenital	• Residual club foot • Arthrogryposis
Traumatic	• Compartment syndrome of the deep posterior compartment • Malunited talar neck fracture
Idiopathic	

CLINICAL PICTURE

- Evaluation of the patients starts with thorough history, including family history of any neurologic problems. Lateral-sided pain is the main complaint. Recurrent ankle sprains can be present.
- Examination of the patient starts with observing their gait. Position of the hindfoot and forefoot is assessed while patient is standing and in seated position. "Peek a boo" sign denoting hindfoot varus can be observed.
- Full neurologic examination including muscle power and reflexes is essential.
- Signs of lateral overload including callosities under the lateral metatarsal heads and stress fractures of the 4th and 5th metatarsals can be present.
- Coleman block test is performed to assess if the hindfoot varus deformity is forefoot driven (**Fig. 7-3**).
- Ankle, subtalar, transverse tarsal, and MTP joints range of motion are carefully assessed.

IMAGING

- AP and lateral standing radiographs of the foot and ankle are usually sufficient.
- AP talo-1st metatarsal angle delineates forefoot adduction.
- Calcaneal pitch and lateral talo-1st metatarsal angle can show hindfoot varus and forefoot plantar flexion, respectively (**Fig. 7-4**).
- Saltzman view can help assess hindfoot alignment.
- Lateral talar tilt and ankle arthritis are detected on AP ankle radiograph.

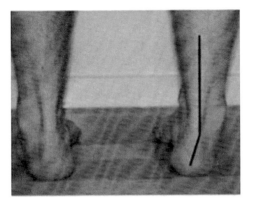

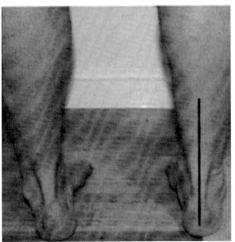

Figure 7-3 Top image showing hindfoot varus deformity on the right. Bottom image showing correction of hindfoot varus with Coleman block test.

- MRI can help detect peroneal (or other tendon) tears and osteochondral lesions.

MANAGEMENT

Conservative Management
- Early, stable, or slowly progressive deformities
- Shoes with wide-toe boxes can be beneficial in metatarsalgia.

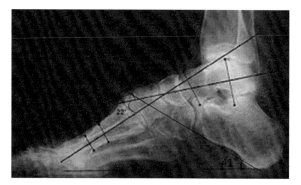

Figure 7-4 Lateral plain radiograph demonstrating + + calcaneal pitch (normal 17°-30°) and lateral talus-1st metatarsal angle of 22° (normal 0° ± 4°).

- Custom-made orthotics with 1st metatarsal head recess, lateral forefoot wedge (*Foot Ankle Int* 2005;26:256)
- Ankle-foot orthosis → patients with severe muscle weakness
- High boot or ankle braces → patients with lateral ankle instability

Surgical Management
General Principles
- Patients vary in presentations so treatment should be individualized.
- Tendon transfer of deforming tendons
- Release of contracted structures
- Realignment osteotomy in the absence of arthritic degenerative changes
- Fusion in fixed deformity with arthritis
- Generally, patients with flexible deformities should undergo joint-preserving surgeries (tendon release and lengthening ± osteotomies), whereas those with fixed deformities will benefit from fusions ± osteotomies.

Soft-Tissue Procedures
- Tight heel cord → TAL versus gastrocnemius recession
- Persistent equinus after heel cord lengthening → ankle and subtalar capsular release
- Midfoot cavus → plantar fascia release
- Tibialis posterior → tibialis anterior and peroneus longus → brevis tendon transfers are the most common out-of-phase transfers performed.
- Several in-phase tendon transfers have been described (eg, EHL → tibialis anterior transfer).

- Claw toes → flexor to extensor tendon transfer
- Hyperextension deformity of MTP of big toe → Jones procedure (+IP fusion)
- Lateral ankle instability → lateral ligament reconstruction (+cavus corrective procedures)

Bony Procedures
- Hindfoot varus that does not correct with a Coleman block test → lateralizing calcaneal osteotomy (*Clin Orthop* 1975;106:254)
- Forefoot-driven hindfoot varus or symptomatic plantarflexed 1st ray → 1st metatarsal dorsiflexion osteotomy
- Midfoot cavus → midfoot dorsiflexion osteotomy
- Residual forefoot adduction → lateral column shortening

Fusion
- Fixed deformity ± arthritis → subtalar, double, or triple arthrodesis
Fixed ankle deformity → ankle fusion + other corrective procedures

STRESS FRACTURES

SHAUN A. KINK • ANNE HOLLY JOHNSON

EPIDEMIOLOGY

- 1% of general population, 15% of runners
- Women > men
- Highest in military recruits, girls' cross-country, girls' gymnastics, boys' cross-country (*AJSM* 2015;43(1):26-33)

PATHOGENESIS

- Submaximal repetitive loading → increased osteoclast activity → increased bone resorption → lagging bone formation → bone fatigues → microfracture → stress fracture
- Stress reaction—bone stress injury due to microfractures
- Stress fracture—coalescence of microfractures into a radiographic fracture line

RISK FACTORS

- **Intrinsic:** Age, sex, bone mineral density, hormonal imbalances, malalignment, poor vascular supply of bone
- **Extrinsic:** Abrupt increase in intensity, duration, or frequency of activity; playing surfaces; improper technique or footwear
- Female athlete triad (eating disorder, amenorrhea, osteoporosis) (*AJSM* 2014;42(4):949-958)

HISTORY AND PE

- Identify any changes in training regimen or equipment
- Elicit medical history (ie, medications, diet, changes in weight, menstrual cycle in females)
- Identify area of tenderness, swelling, and overall alignment of the extremity

IMAGING

- **Radiographs:** Initial (85%) and follow-up (50%) are often negative.
- **Bone scintigraphy:** Three-phase bone scan—high sensitivity, poor specificity

- MRI—gold standard—high sensitivity, high specificity—additionally able to evaluate surrounding soft tissue
- CT scan—best for identifying fracture lines, areas of sclerosis, and comminution

MEDIAL MALLEOLUS STRESS FRACTURES

- Most common in running and jumping athletes
- Repetitive torsional loads placed on the medial malleolus, some new literature implicating anterior ankle impingement
- Complaint of vague anterior medial ankle pain with activity, TTP along the medial malleolus, swelling present
- **Fracture pattern:** Oblique or vertical fxr line from medial plafond to medial cortex
- **DDx:** Posterior tibialis tendonitis, deltoid ligament injuries, ankle arthritis, anterior ankle impingement, tarsal tunnel syndrome
- **Work-up:** Radiographs (70% negative). MRI ~100% sensitive, CT scan to characterize fracture pattern
- **Treatment:** Nonoperative: short period of immobilization → gradual return to activity after pain subsides → return to play 6 to 8 weeks
- **Operative treatment:** Percutaneous screw fixation, ORIF with screw or plate constructs → return to weight bearing 1 to 3 weeks post-op
- Successful treatment has been achieved with surgical and conservative measures.
- Surgical fixation may allow earlier return to sports (2.4 vs 7.6 weeks) (*Sports Health* 2014;6(6):527-530).

NAVICULAR STRESS FRACTURES

- High-risk sports include track and field, football, rugby, and basketball.
- Tenuous blood supply indicated in pathogenesis → anterior tibial and posterior tibial supply navicular → central 1/3 is watershed area
- Short 1st MT and long 2nd MT also implicated → increased torsional load transmitted to central 1/3 of navicular
- **Fracture pattern:** Dorsal proximal to distal lateral
- Complains of vague dorsal medial foot pain, TTP along the N spot (dorsal proximal navicular)
- **Work-up:** X-rays (rarely helpful), MRI, or bone scan to diagnose, CT scan to characterize fracture

- **Treatment:** NWB cast for 6 to 8 weeks (WB cast worse outcomes) → resume activity once no TTP at N spot
- **Surgical treatment indications:** Displaced fractures, complete nondisplaced fracture with sclerosis, failed 3 months conservative treatment
- Treatment with 2 to 3 4.0 or 4.5 partially threaded screws from lateral to medial and 6 to 8 weeks NWB

5TH METATARSAL STRESS FRACTURES

- Most common in football, basketball, and soccer players
- Tenuous blood supply to proximal metadiaphysis
- Complains of history of pain with abrupt worsening of symptoms
- Fractures ~1.5 cm distal to base have less predictable healing → 25% require surgical intervention
- Torg classification (*JBJS* 1984;66(2):209-214): Type I → acute fracture, narrow fracture line, no intramedullary sclerosis; Type II → delayed union, wide fracture line, intramedullary sclerosis; Type III → nonunion, complete obliteration of intramedullary canal by sclerotic bone
- **Torg I fracture:** 6 to 8 weeks NWB cast immobilization → Return to pre-injury activity ~12 weeks
- **Torg II and III fracture:** Surgical intervention with intramedullary screw or plate fixation, curettage, and bone grafting

Type	Fracture	X-ray Findings	Treatment
Torg I	Acute fracture	Narrow fracture line, no intramedullary sclerosis	6–8 wk NWB in cast
Torg II	Delayed union	Wide fracture line, intramedullary sclerosis	ORIF, bone graft
Torg III	Nonunion	Complete obliteration of intramedullary canal by sclerotic bone	ORIF, bone graft

ARTHROSCOPY PRINCIPLES

SHAUN A. KINK • ANNE HOLLY JOHNSON

ARTHROSCOPY OF ANKLE

INDICATIONS FOR SUPINE ANKLE ARTHROSCOPY

- Soft-tissue injury and impingement
- Bony impingement
- Arthrofibrosis
- Instability
- Aid with fracture reduction
- Synovitis
- Biopsy of intra-articular soft tissues
- Loose bodies
- End-stage arthritis requiring fusion
- Unexplained pain/swelling
- Mechanical symptoms (locking, catching, painful popping)
- Osteochondral injuries

INDICATIONS FOR PRONE POSTERIOR ANKLE/ HINDFOOT ARTHROSCOPY

- Loose bodies, ossicles, posttraumatic calcifications, avulsion fragments, and osteophytes along posterior tibial rim or level of subtalar joint
- Chondromatosis; posterior talar/tibial/calcaneal osteochondral defects; degenerative joint changes
- Posttraumatic synovitis, villonodular synovitis, and syndesmotic soft-tissue impingement
- Posterior ankle impingement → hypertrophic posterior talar process, os trigonum, talus bipartita
- Avulsions fragments and posttraumatic calcifications in deep portion of deltoid ligament
- FHL tendinopathy
- Recurrent peroneal tendon dislocation

CONTRAINDICATIONS

- Localized soft-tissue infection → prevent potential intra-articular dissemination of cellulitis or soft-tissue abscess

- Severe ankle arthritis not amenable to arthroscopic arthrodesis (ie, significant deformity or stiffness)
- General medical conditions precluding surgical intervention

EQUIPMENT

- Video arthroscopes → 1.9- and 2.7-mm arthroscopes most commonly used, 4.0-mm may be used in specific situations (ie, ankle fusion) → smaller scopes allow improved maneuverability, decreased instrument crowding, and decreased inadvertent chondral damage, at the risk of increased choice of instrument bending and breakage
- Instruments → small joint instruments preferred → 2.0-, 2.9-, 3.5-mm shavers and burrs; 3.5- and 4.5-mm ring and cup curettes; 1.5-mm probes; 2.9- and 3.5-mm graspers and baskets; microfracture picks
- Ankle distractors → both invasive and noninvasive exist → invasive use pins within tibia, talus, and/or calcaneus to obtain distraction and have risks of infection, NV injury, fracture, wound issues → noninvasive distractors (ie, manual distraction, gravity distraction, or controlled strap distraction devices) are preferred as they have fewer complications than invasive techniques → distraction force should be limited to <30 lb for <1 hour (*Arthroscopy* 1996;12:64-69)

POSITIONING AND PREPARATION

- Supine → thigh holder placed superior to popliteal fossa (minimize pressure in popliteal fossa) with hip at approx 45 to 50 degrees of flexion → tourniquet placed on thigh (may or may not inflate) → ipsilateral thigh post can be used to help maintain foot and ankle position → pad all bony prominences to prevent NV compromise secondary to pressure
- Prone → patient placed in prone position with foot off end of bed to allow dorsiflexion → triangular bump can be used under shin → thigh tourniquet is placed → ipsilateral thigh post can be used to maintain position

ARTHROSCOPY PUMPS

- Help to maintain hemostasis, improve visualization, and allow intra-op adjustments to be made → risk of extravasation of fluid into foot or anterolateral compartment causing increased compartmental pressure

ANESTHESIA

- General anesthesia with complete paralysis facilitates distraction → regional block (ie, popliteal block) can be used as well to aid in postoperative pain relief → additional saphenous local anesthesia may be required

ARTHROSCOPIC ANKLE PORTALS

- Anteromedial portal → placed just medial to the tibialis anterior tendon at the level of the joint → saphenous nerve and vein at risk
- Anterolateral portal → placed just lateral to the peroneus tertius tendon at the level of the joint → superficial peroneal nerve at risk
- Anterocentral and medial midline portals are described but rarely used due to significant risk of NV structures and limited utility.
- Posteromedial portal → placed just medial to Achilles tendon → FHL, FDL, tibial nerve, and posterior tibial artery at risk
- Posterolateral portal → placed just lateral to Achilles tendon at the level of the tip of the fibula → Sural nerve and small saphenous vein at risk
- Trans-Achilles portal is described but risks damage to Achilles tendon and reduced mobility thus rarely used.
- **Complications:** NV injury make up 49% of ankle arthroscopy complications (*Arthroscopy* 1996;12:200-208) → attributed to portal and distractor pin placement; wound complications

SUBTALAR ARTHROSCOPY

- Equipment, positioning, pumps, and anesthesia are similar to that used in ankle arthroscopy.
- Can be done with patient in supine, lateral, or prone position → prone positioning utilizes posterolateral and posteromedial portals
- Supine and lateral utilized lateral subtalar portals as described below.

INDICATIONS FOR SUBTALAR ARTHROSCOPY

- Pain, swelling, stiffness, and locking within subtalar joint nonresponsive to conservative measures
- Os trigonum
- Loose bodies
- Synovitis
- Sinus tarsi syndrome
- Posteromedial talar facet fracture
- Osteochondral lesions
- Subfibular pain, status post-calcaneal fracture
- Tarsal coalitions
- Subtalar arthrodesis

SUBTALAR LATERAL PORTAL PLACEMENT

- Anterolateral portal → 2.5 to 3 cm anterior to fibula superior to central portal
- Central portal (middle portal) → one thumb's breadth anterior and inferior to the tip of the fibula
- Posterolateral portal → lateral to the Achilles tendon at the level of the tip of the fibula
- Structures at risk with these portals are the peroneal tendons, sural nerve, and small saphenous vein.

OSTEOCHONDRAL LESIONS OF TALUS

SHAUN A. KINK • ANNE HOLLY JOHNSON

PATHOGENESIS

- Majority of talar OLTs are secondary to trauma, minority secondary to local ischemic changes and necrosis (usually medial).
- Medial lesions are the most common → mid to posteromedial lesions → d/t compression fracture of subchondral bone
- Lateral lesions → mid to anterolateral lesions → d/t sheer stresses seen at the time of injury

CHARACTERISTICS

- **Medial lesion:** larger, deeper, more commonly cystic and chronic
- **Lateral lesions:** smaller, shallow, more commonly displaced, symptomatic, and acute

CLINICAL PRESENTATION AND EXAM

- History of inversion sprain → continued pain after 6 to 8 weeks
- Pain worse during or after loading or exercise.
- Persistent swelling and stiffness
- Locking, clicking, catching → displaced fragment
- Effusion, TTP along talar dome

IMAGING

- Radiographs → lucencies along talar dome, associated injuries/avulsions, loose bodies/fragments
- **MRI:** Gold standard for diagnosis → 3 T more sensitive for diagnosis → identify break in subchondral bone plate
- **CT:** Useful to evaluate size of lesion and cystic components

Classifications

Berndt and Harty Radiographic Classification	
Stage 1	Small area of subchondral compression
Stage 2	Partial fragment detachment
Stage 3	Complete fragment detachment but not displaced
Stage 4	Displaced fragment

Ferkel and Sgaglione CT Staging System	
Stage I	Cystic lesion within dome of talus with an intact roof on all views
Stage 2a	Cystic lesion communication to talar dome surface
Stage 2b	Open articular surface lesion with overlying nondisplaced fragment
Stage 3	Nondisplaced lesion with lucency
Stage 4	Displaced fragment

MRI Staging System	
Stage I	Subchondral trabecular compression, marrow edema
Stage 2a	Formation of subchondral cyst
Stage 2	Incomplete separation of fragment
Stage 3	Unattached, undisplaced fragment, synovial fluid surrounding fragment
Stage 4	Displaced fragment

NONOPERATIVE TREATMENT

- Contraindicated in acute displaced lesions
- Consists of varying degrees of immobilization → cast versus boot → NWB versus WBAT in supportive device → 2 to 4 weeks duration
- Activity modifications, NSAIDs, bracing, corticosteroid injections

OPERATIVE TREATMENT

- Failed conservative treatment of 3 to 6 months and acute displaced fragments
- **Bone marrow stimulation (BMS):** Debridement of OLT to obtain stable cartilage margins → penetrate subchondral bone → egress of bone marrow cells → formation of fibrocartilage surface
- **BMS:** Transtalar or transmalleolar drilling: requires stable cartilaginous cap → K-wires used to drill retrograde or antegrade into lesion → develop vascular channels → stimulate healing of subchondral bone; retrograde bone grafting can be performed as well
- **Cartilage restoration: Osteochondral autograft transfer (OATs):** Debridement of OLT to stable margins → measure defect → obtain osteochondral plug (typically from non–weight-bearing portion of knee) → insert plug in OLT

- **Cartilage restoration: Osteochondral allograft transfer:** Require CT scan for talar dimensions → bone bank obtains match → implantation within 14 days d/t chondrocyte viability; can be used for both small and, in particular, large cavitary defects (ie, shell allografts)
- **Cartilage restoration: Autologous cartilage implantation:** Two procedures needed: first procedure → harvest chondrocytes from knee or margin of OLT lesion → lab cultures chondrocytes (~2-3 weeks) second procedure → periosteal flap placed over OLT → cultured chondrocytes injected under flap
- **Cartilage restoration:** Particulated juvenile cartilage → debride lesions → bone graft cystic areas → place cartilage over lesion → secure with fibrin glue
- **Adjuvants to microfracture:** Cartilage extracellular matrix allograft

---

TREATMENT CONSIDERATIONS

- **Size:** Lesions >1.5 cm² poorer outcomes with microfracture
- **Cystic lesions:** Often require bone grafting (calcaneal or tibial), OATs, or allograft transfer
- **Containment:** Uncontained shoulder lesions may not fare as well with microfracture

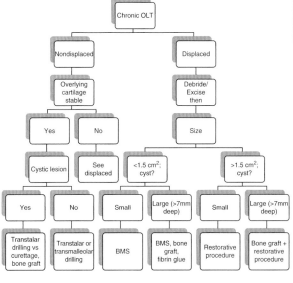

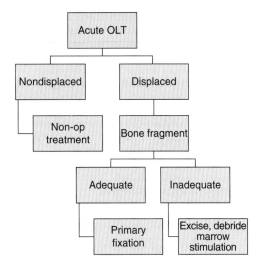

- Previous treatments
- Stability of cartilaginous cap
- **Acute versus chronic lesion:** Acute displaced lesions →
  ORIF if adequate subchondral bone still attached; chronic
  lesions → excise, debride, treatment options as discussed
  above

SUGGESTED READINGS

Hahn DB, Aanstoos ME, Wilkins RM. Osteochondral lesions
of the talus with fresh talar allografts. *Foot Ankle Int.*
2010;31(4):277-282.

Wodicka R, Ferkel E, Ferkel R. Osteochondral lesions of the
ankle. *Foot Ankle Int.* 2016;37(9):1023-1034.

Woelfle JV, Reichel H, Javaheripour-Otto K, et al. Clinical
outcome and magnetic resonance imaging after
osteochondral autologous transplantation in osteochondritis
dissecans of the talus. *Foot Ankle Int.* 2013;34(2):173-179.

ACHILLES TENDON RUPTURES

SHAUN A. KINK • ANNE HOLLY JOHNSON

ANATOMY

- Gastrocnemius-soleus complex (triceps surae) crosses both the ankle and the knee → innervated by the tibial nerve → consolidates into the Achilles tendon → composed of gastrocnemius muscle, which originates on the posterior femoral condyles, and soleus, which originates on the posterior aspect of the tibia, fibula, and interosseous membrane → Achilles tendon inserts broadly on calcaneal tuberosity
- Gastrocnemius is a powerful plantar flexor of ankle with knee extended → soleus is more powerful with knee flexed
- Two bursae exist → retrocalcaneal bursa between Achilles tendon and calcaneus → Achilles bursa between Achilles tendon and skin
- Achilles tendon is surrounded by paratenon but no true synovial sheath
- Vascular supply → proximal intramuscular arterial branches → distally through interosseous arterioles from calcaneus → zone of relative avascularity 2 to 6 cm proximal to calcaneal insertion → zone is more susceptible to degenerative changes

ETIOLOGY

- Direct injuries → posterior ankle crush injuries or lacerations
- Indirect injuries → overriding theme is rapid loading process on already tensed tendon: (1) sharp unexpected dorsiflexion force to ankle coupled with strong contracture of triceps surae; (2) pushing off weight-bearing foot with knee in extension; (3) strong dorsiflexion force on a plantar-flexed ankle
- Peak occurrence in third to fifth decade; 5:1 M:F ratio; recreational athletes; occur within 2 to 6 cm of calcaneal insertion
- **RF:** Fluoroquinolone antibiotic use, corticosteroid use, corticosteroid injections, genetic predisposition (26% risk of contralateral rupture of Achilles) (*Disord Foot Ankle* 1991:2355-2360), intrinsic degenerative changes within tendon
- Location of tears: middle portion (72%-73%); proximal muscu-lotendinous junction (4%-14%); distal ruptures (14%-24%)

HISTORY AND PHYSICAL EXAM

- Hx of misstep, jump, or push off → sensation of snap or audible pop followed by acute pain, difficulty walking, weak plantar flexion → reports sensation of getting kicked or struck in posterior heel region
- PE shows palpable defect in Achilles tendon with diminished plantar flexion strength → ecchymosis and swelling → increased resting dorsiflexion compared to contralateral side → +Thompson test (patient prone with knee flexed to 90°, squeeze calf, lack of plantar flexion of foot is a positive test indicating Achilles rupture) → +Matles test (patient prone with knee flexed 90°, increased dorsiflexion to uninjured side is a positive test indicating Achilles rupture)
- Plantar flexion strength may be present but decreased secondary to recruitment of other plantar flexors and intact plantaris muscle.

RADIOGRAPHIC EXAMINATION

- **X-rays:** Identify avulsion fractures, intra-substance calcifications, disruption in Kager triangle
- **Ultrasound:** Visualize tendon rupture, internal structure of tendon, ability to appose ruptured ends dynamically, operator dependent
- **MRI:** Visualize tendon rupture, internal structure of tendon, retrocalcaneal pathologies, more valuable in chronic ruptures

CONSERVATIVE TREATMENT

- **Pros:** Decreased medical costs, lower morbidity, no surgical risks (ie, wound complications, anesthetic complications)
- **Cons:** Risk of reduced strength and endurance if healed elongated, higher re-rupture risk
- Cast immobilization being replaced by short-term splinting followed by early rehabilitation
- Early rehab has shown lower risk of re-rupture than cast immobilization.
- Chronic ruptures can be treated non-op with rocker bottom shoes, rigid AFO, or ground reaction AFO → reserved for low demand or high surgical risk patients → non-op results inferior to surgically managed chronic Achilles tendon ruptures (Christensen et al. *Acta Chir Scand* 1953;106:50-60)

SURGICAL TREATMENT

- **Acute ruptures:** Various methods including open repair, mini-open repair, and percutaneous methods of repair → open repair and mini-open have shown similar results → mini-open and percutaneous thought to lower surgical wound complications but may have higher rate of sural nerve injuries
- **Chronic ruptures:** Treatment depends on ability to re-approximate tendon ends (more difficult in chronic setting) and gap after adequate debridement of tendon → treatment consists of repair, augmentation, or reconstruction
- **Repair chronic tendons:** Able to re-approximate tension ends or tendon healed in elongated fashion → Z-shortening of tendon → reestablish resting tendon and function
- **Reconstruction:** Method depends on gap size: 3 to 5 cm: V-Y advancement ± augmentation (turn down flaps) or tendon augmentation (plantaris, FHL, FDL, peroneus brevis, gracilis, semi-T, synthetic material); >5 cm: Tendon transfer (FHL, FDL, or PB) or reconstruction with gracilis, semi-T, or fascia lata tendon. Large defects not amendable to tendon transfer → reconstruct with Achilles allograft
- Wound healing and infection are significant risks when proceeding with surgical intervention → wound complications in this area can be devastating and difficult to treat → may require wound VAC treatments or free tissue transfers
- Surgical complications → incidence of 20% → include keloid formation, sural nerve injuries, adhesions, infection, skin slough, and re-rupture (*Clin Orthop Relat Res* 1986;207:156-163)

ACHILLES TENDINOPATHY

SHAUN A. KINK • ANNE HOLLY JOHNSON

ANATOMY

- Gastrocnemius-soleus complex (triceps surae) transverses both the ankle and the knee → innervated by the tibial nerve → consolidates into the Achilles tendon → composed of the gastrocnemius muscle, which originates on the posterior femoral condyles and soleus which originates on the posterior aspect of the tibia, fibula, and interosseous membrane → Achilles tendon inserts broadly on calcaneal tuberosity
- Gastrocnemius is a powerful plantar flexor of ankle with knee extended → soleus is more powerful with knee flexed
- Two bursae exist → retrocalcaneal bursa between Achilles tendon and calcaneus → Achilles bursa between Achilles tendon and skin
- Achilles tendon is surrounded by paratenon but no true synovial sheath.
- Vascular supply → proximal intramuscular arterial branches → distally through interosseous arterioles from calcaneus → zone of relative avascularity 2 to 6 cm proximal to calcaneal insertion → more susceptible to degenerative changes

CLASSIFICATION

- **Duration of symptoms:** Acute → less than 3 weeks; subacute → 3 to 6 weeks; chronic → greater than 6 weeks of symptoms
- **Location of symptoms:** Insertional tendonitis → occurs at or around the insertion of the Achilles on the calcaneus, ±Haglund deformity, ±calcaneal spur within tendon; noninsertional tendonitis → occurs proximal to the insertion
- **Stages of inflammation:** Stage 1—Paratenonitis → inflammatory changes localized to paratenon, tendon appears normal, + fluid and thickening of paratenon, ±adhesions to tendon. Stage 2—Paratenonitis with tendinosis, tendon becomes nodular and thickened, + inflammation within the paratenon. Stage 3—Tendinosis, degenerative changes within tendon without inflammation of the paratenon

Stage 1	Paratenonitis	• Inflammatory changes within paratenon (thick, fluid) • Tendon normal • ±Adhesions
Stage 2	Paratenonitis with tendinosis	• Inflammatory changes within paratenon • Nodular thickening of tendon
Stage 3	Tendinosis	• No inflammation of paratenon • Degenerative changes to tendon

HISTORY AND PHYSICAL EXAM

- **Patients describe:**
  - Pain with initial activity that increases with exercise
  - Transient pain with running in early stages
  - Pain that may progress to pain with walking or even rest
- Haglund deformity ("pump bump") characterized by posterolateral prominence of calcaneus, pain with constricting footwear or closely contoured heel counter
- **Pain location (*Am J Sports Med* 1988;16(6):616-628):**
  - Mid-tendon (51%)
  - Tendon insertion (24%)
  - Proximal tendon (10%)
  - Diffusely (15%)
- Paratenonitis displays tenderness and swelling that remains fixed with active ROM; tendinosis displays an area of tenderness that moves with active ROM (painful arc sign)
- Retrocalcaneal bursitis → pain elicited just anterior to Achilles, two-finger squeeze test produces pain by squeezing medial to lateral at a location superior and anterior to tendon insertion
- Palpation of tendon and Thompson test performed to exclude tendon rupture

RADIOGRAPHIC EXAMINATION

- X-rays—identify calcifications within the tendon, insertional calcifications, Haglund deformity magnitude using parallel pitch lines as described by Pavlov (*Radiology* 1982;144(1):83-88)
- Ultrasound—can identify partial Achilles tears, paratenon thickening, tendinosis, nodularity, cystic changes, or calcifications
- MRI—provides similar data to ultrasound but can also evaluate other causes of posterior ankle pain

TENDINOPATHY 8-18

CONSERVATIVE TREATMENT

- NSAIDs, rest, immobilization, activity modifications, and stretching are the mainstays of conservative treatment.
- Heel lifts and night splints can be incorporated into treatment regimens.
- Brisement (injections of local anesthetic or saline) into the pseudosheath can be used in paratenonitis when adhesions are present.
- Eccentric stretching and strengthening has been shown to provide high patient satisfaction, reduced pain, and successful return to activity levels (*FAI* 2011;32:843-849).
- Extracorporeal shock wave therapy → reduces inflammation, improves blood flow → shown to be an effective adjuvant in both insertional and noninsertional tendonitis (*JBJS* 2008;90:52-61)
- Recommend at least 3 to 6 months of conservative treatment prior to surgical intervention

SURGICAL TREATMENT

- Appropriate surgical procedure depends on the location of tendonitis, presence of Haglund deformity, degree of tendon involvement.
- Insertional tendonitis ± Haglund → debridement of degenerative tissue, excision of retrocalcaneal bursa, excision of Haglund deformity, repair or supplementation of tendon if necessary → lateral approach or tendon-splitting approach can be used → >50% of tendon debrided consider tendon transfer such as FHL, FDL, peroneal brevis
- Arthroscopic debridement of insertional tendonitis → able to debride bursa and Haglund deformity → unable to significantly debride tendon → useful when MRI does not show significant tendinosis
- Noninsertional → debridement of inflammatory paratenon tissue → takedown of any adhesions present → longitudinal debridement of degenerative areas of tendon → repair with tubularization of tendon if <50% → >50% debrided supplementation with FHL or FDL
- Gastrocnemius recession has shown success in the treatment of noninsertional Achilles tendonitis (*FAI* 2013;34:481-485).

PERONEAL TENDON DISORDERS

SHAUN A. KINK • ANNE HOLLY JOHNSON

ANATOMY

- Peroneus longus (PL) → originates on the lateral condyle of tibia and head and midlateral aspect of the fibula → inserts on the inferior aspect of the 1st metatarsal and cuneiform → innervated by the superficial peroneal nerve (SPN) → acts to plantar flex and evert the foot, plantar flex 1st metatarsal → runs posterior to the peroneus brevis at the level of the distal fibula, below the peroneal tubercle, through the cuboid tunnel and across the foot to the 1st metatarsal → avascular regions of the tendon occur as tendon courses around the lateral malleolus and the cuboid
- Peroneus brevis (PB) → originates on the midportion of the lateral fibula → inserts on the base of the 5th metatarsal → innervated by the SPN → acts to evert and plantar flex the foot → runs anterior to the longus at the level of the distal fibula, superior to the peroneal tubercle → avascular area as tendon courses around the lateral malleolus
- Os peroneum → accessory ossicle located within the PL along the lateral aspect of the cuboid
- Sural nerve → located just posterior to the tendons above the level of the distal fibula → crosses over tendons between 1 and 2 cm from the calcaneocuboid joint

PERONEAL TENOSYNOVITIS

History and Physical Exam
- Pain at posterolateral aspect of hindfoot, worsens with activity, diminished by rest → may recall history of traumatic episode (inversion injury) followed by onset of pain
- Pain with palpation along the course of the peroneal tendons, resisted eversion, passive inversion of foot
- Prominent peroneal tubercle may be palpated.
- May have a history of fibula or calcaneal fracture

Radiographic Examination
- X-rays → identify calcaneal fractures, avulsion injuries, prominent peroneal tubercle, presence of os peroneum, evaluate alignment of the foot and the ankle
- MRI → identify tenosynovitis (abnormal fluid within tendon sheath), longitudinal tears of the peroneal tendons, and

complete disruptions → helpful to identify other causes of lateral ankle pathology → magic angle effect may increase false positive results

- Ultrasound → can evaluate tendon tears/disruptions, tenosynovitis around the tendons → provides dynamic aspect of exam to help identify subluxations/dislocations of tendons

Conservative Treatment
- NSAIDs, activity modifications, immobilization in cast/CAM boot for 3 to 4 weeks, and physical therapy
- Causative factors may be sudden change in training regimen, training surface, or intensity/duration of training → alterations in training regimen will allow resolution of symptoms

Surgical Treatment
- Tenosynovectomy (open or tendoscopic) → inspect tendons for tears → debride synovial tissue, excise prominent peroneal tubercle → excise os peroneum if enlarged, irregular, or damaged → repair superior peroneal retinaculum if needed

---

PERONEAL TENDON TEARS

Etiology
- PB tendon tears are more common than longus tears → PB tears typically located behind the lateral malleolus → PL tears located at the peroneal tubercle or os peroneum
- PB tears → mechanical disruption within the fibular groove → plantar flexion (15°-25°) and inversion → associated with chronic subluxation of tendons, peroneus quartus tendon, overcrowding within peroneal tendon sheath (low-lying muscle belly, tenosynovitis)
- PL tears → associated with hypertrophy of peroneal tubercle and presence of os peroneum
- Chronic lateral ankle instability → repetitive injury to peroneal tendons with each subsequent sprain → attritional tears of peroneal tendons
- Hindfoot varus → recurrent sprains often seen with hindfoot varus → attritional tears of peroneal tendons

History and Physical Exam
- Pain at the posterolateral aspect of the hindfoot, worsens with activity, diminished by rest → may recall history of traumatic episode (inversion injury) followed by onset of pain
- Recalcitrant synovitis and swelling along tendons, weakness, fatigue, and ankle instability → pain with resisted eversion or passive inversion

- PB tears → pain typically located retromalleolar
- PL tears → pain along peroneal tubercle or cuboid notch/os peroneum
- Positive peroneal compression test—knee flexed 90°, foot and ankle relaxed plantar-flexed position, examiner's thumb over superior retinaculum, patient forcibly everts and dorsiflexes foot → pain, crepitation, and popping → + test
- Bupivacaine injections within tendon sheath may aid in diagnosis → sensitivity decreased by connections with ankle and subtalar joints in 15% of patients
- Evaluate all patients for lateral ankle instability, hindfoot varus

Radiographic Examination
- **X-rays:** Evaluate for os peroneum retraction/fragmentation/fracture, hypertrophied peroneal tubercle, hindfoot varus, avulsion injuries/previous trauma
- **MRI:** Evaluates for peroneal tendon tears, nondisplaced os peroneum fractures, additional lateral ankle pathology → magic angle effect increase false positive results
- **Ultrasound:** Useful in identifying tears and dynamic instability of tears → sensitivity is operator dependent

Conservative Treatment
- NSAIDs, activity modifications, rest, immobilization in cast/CAM boot 3 to 4 weeks, and physical therapy
- Ankle brace to limit inversion and eversion
- Lateral heel wedges or orthotics to correct foot malalignment

Surgical Treatment
- Debridement of longitudinal tears and repair of the tendon
- Non-repairable tendons can be treated in various ways → tenodesis of damaged tendon to intact tendon → allograft or autograft tendon grafting → tendon transfers
- Tendon transfers should be utilized in the event of significant atrophy of muscle and limited excursion of tendon
- Must identify and treat concomitant ankle instability and malalignment

PERONEAL TENDON SUBLUXATION-DISLOCATION

Anatomy
- Fibular groove → typically concave in 82% of patients → 18% can have convex or flat fibular grooves → predisposing to peroneal instability

- Superior peroneal retinaculum → distal 2 cm of fibula → confluence of distal calf fascia and peroneal sheath → attaches to posterolateral fibula and calcaneus or Achilles tendon sheath or both
- Fibular ridge with fibrocartilaginous cap provides fibular groove with additional depth of 2 to 4 mm.
- Inferior peroneal retinaculum → originates and inserts on calcaneus just below the sinus tarsi → no role in stability of peroneals at the level of the ankle

Mechanism of Injury
- Forceful dorsiflexion and inversion injury to ankle → disruption of the SPR → dislocation of the peroneal tendons
- Chronic subluxation seen with recurrent ankle sprains → leading to attenuation of SPR → loss of constraint to peroneal tendons
- Neuromuscular abnormalities (paralysis, polio) have been associated with peroneal tendon dislocations.

Classification
- Grade 1 (51%)—SPR elevated off lateral malleolus, tendons lying between bone and periosteum
- Grade 2 (33%)—Fibrocartilage ridge elevated off fibula, tendons lying beneath ridge
- Grade 3 (16%)—Cortical avulsion from fibula, tendons beneath fibular fragment (*JBJS* 1976;58:670-672)

History and Physical Examination
- Acute dislocations → trauma, inversion sprain → pain at retromalleolar area
- Complain of snapping and popping or instability on uneven ground
- Subluxation with movement of foot from a plantar-flexed, inverted position to dorsiflexed and everted position
- Evaluate for coexisting lateral ankle instability

Radiographic Examination
- **X-rays:** Avulsion off fibular cortex
- **CT scan:** Evaluate configuration of the fibular groove
- **MRI:** Evaluate concomitant peroneal tendon injury and SPR
- **Ultrasound:** Dynamic exam to identify subluxation/dislocation

Conservative Treatment
- Acute dislocations can be initially treated with a short leg cast for 5 to 6 weeks.
- Success rate is <50% (*JBJS* 1976;58:670-672).

Surgical Treatment

- Treatment is geared toward addressing all issues predisposing patient to dislocations
  - SPR repair $\pm$ augmentation—suture anchors or suture repair through osseous tunnels, augmentation with Achilles, PB, plantaris, or allograft
  - Excision of low-lying muscle belly
  - Fibular groove deepening osteotomy for flat or convex fibular grooves
  - Address peroneal pathology—tears/tenosynovitis more common in chronic tears

ANTERIOR TIBIAL TENDINOPATHY

SHAUN A. KINK • ANNE HOLLY JOHNSON

ANATOMY

- Anterior tibialis tendon → originates in the proximal half of the anterior tibia and interosseous membrane → inserts on the plantar medial 1st cuneiform and 1st metatarsal base → innervated by the deep peroneal nerve → dorsiflexes and inverts foot → avascular zone where tendon runs under the superior and inferior retinacula

ANTERIOR TIBIALIS TENDONITIS

History and Physical Examination
- Patients describe a burning pain, located along the medial midfoot, dorsomedial swelling, pain with activity and at night.
- Tenderness to palpation along the AT tendon and insertion
- Tibialis anterior passive stretch test—performed by plantar flexion, hindfoot eversion, midfoot abduction, and pronation force on foot → positive if reproduces pain
- Pain with resisted dorsiflexion, unable to walk on heel, +Silfverskiold test

Radiographic Examination
- X-rays → identify soft-tissue swelling, alignment of foot, and presence of midfoot arthritis
- MRI → identify tendon thickening/degeneration, peritendon edema and synovitis, increased signal/edema within tendon insertion → identify longitudinal tears → additional midfoot pathology
- Ultrasound → identify presence of synovitis, thickening/degeneration, longitudinal tears

Conservative Treatment
- NSAIDs, activity modification (avoid inclines and declines), immobilization in cast/CAM boot for 3 to 4 weeks, physical therapy, and custom full-length accommodative medial longitudinal arch support orthosis.

Surgical Treatment
- Insertional AT tendonitis → debridement of attachment and repair to medial cuneiform
- Longitudinal tears → require debridement and repair → consider augmentation with EHL tendon transfer especially with <50% AT tendon post-debridement → risk of spontaneous rupture after repair (*FAI* 2010;31:212-219)

ANTERIOR TIBIALIS TENDON RUPTURES

History and Physical Examination
- Acute traumatic ruptures → episode of forced excessive plantar flexion against a contracted AT tendon → pain along AT tendon/anterior ankle
- Acute on chronic ruptures → often attritional ruptures/degenerative tears secondary to inflammatory arthritis, gout, RA, impingement from underlying exostosis, local steroid injection → most common in men 50 to 70 y/o → no antecedent trauma → seek medical attention months later for foot drop
- Patient complaint → acute ruptures of pain and loss of dorsiflexion strength → chronic ruptures of catching toes/tripping while walking
- Exam → weak dorsiflexion, inability to walk on heels → palpable defect in AT tendon → palpable mass along anterior ankle → recruitment of EHL/EDL for dorsiflexion → steppage gait
- Rule out peroneal nerve palsy or L4 to L5 radiculopathy as cause.

Radiographic Examination
- X-rays → identify exostosis involved in attritional ruptures
- MRI → identify tendon rupture and location of retracted ends → evaluate tendon for degenerative changes → identify additional pathology
- Ultrasound → identify tendon rupture and location of retracted ends → evaluate tendon for degenerative changes

Conservative Treatment
- Acute ruptures → surgical treatment often recommended, especially high-demand patients → conservative treatment in elderly, low-demand, medically unfit for surgery patients
- Chronic ruptures → consideration of patient demands and activity

- Treatment consists of bracing with various AFOs (Allard, Posterior Leaf Spring AFO, double upright brace) to improve ambulation and improve activity level.

Surgical Treatment
- Acute ruptures → direct repair of tendon → reinsertion to medial cuneiform in distal tears/avulsion tears
- Chronic ruptures → retraction and scarring may inhibit end to end repair → require hamstring allograft/autograft reconstruction to bridge gap or sliding advancement/turn down or EHL transfer
- Must recognize presence of Achilles tendon contracture in delayed treatment → aggressive stretching preoperatively → may require Achilles lengthening or gastrocnemius recession

ANKLE FRACTURES

TONYA L. DIXON • DANIEL GUSS • NASEF MOHAMED NASEF

ANATOMY

- The ankle is a modified hinge joint.
- Unlike most joints, its articulation consists of three bones rather than two: the tibia and fibula above, and the talus below.
- During ankle dorsiflexion, the talus externally rotates 5° and slides posteriorly; the directions reverse during ankle plantar flexion.
- Ankle dorsiflexion is coupled with subtalar joint eversion, whereas ankle plantar flexion is coupled with subtalar joint inversion.
- The medial (deltoid) and lateral (lateral collateral) ligaments are critically important to underlying ankle stability because they collectively maintain normal relationship and function between these three bones.
- Injury is often due to twisting (rotation) or direct axial loading (impaction); sometimes due to eversion (abduction) or inversion (adduction).

Common Classifications	
Lauge-Hansen	
Supination External Rotation	
Type 1	AITFL rupture w/wo avulsion fracture (fx)
Type 2	Lateral malleolus fx—spiral; usually at or just above joint line
Type 3	PITFL rupture or posterior malleolus fx
Type 4	Deep deltoid tear or medial malleolus fx (transverse)
Pronation External Rotation	
Type 1	Deep deltoid tear or medial malleolus fx (transverse)
Type 2	AITFL rupture w/wo avulsion fx
Type 3	Lateral malleolus fx (spiral)—runs anterosuperior to posteroinferior; usually occurs higher up leg
Type 4	PITFL or lateral posterior malleolus fx
Supination Adduction	
Type 1	Transverse, avulsion fibular fx
Type 2	Medial malleolus fx, vertical sheer
	Anteromedial tibial comminution/impaction
Pronation Abduction	
Type 1	Medial malleolus fx (transverse) or rupture of deltoid ligament
Type 2	Syndesmosis rupture
Type 3	Transverse or short oblique fx of lateral malleolus at or above syndesmosis

First word designates foot position and second word designates direction of deforming force.

Anatomic Classification
- Isolated medial malleolus
- Isolated lateral malleolus
- Bimalleolar
- Trimalleolar
- Pilon (higher energy distal tibial metaphyseal fracture ± intra-articular extension, ± fibular fracture)

Danis-Weber (Based on Location of Fibular Fracture)
- A—Infratectal or infrasyndesmotic (below level of joint line)
- B—Transtectal or transsyndesmotic (at level of joint line)
- C—Supratectal or suprasyndesmotic (above level of joint line)

DIAGNOSIS

- Physical examination—deformity, soft-tissue compromise, neurovascular status, swelling
- Radiographs—AP, mortise, lateral
- Weight-bearing views can help determine ankle fracture stability if patient can tolerate
- External rotation stress view can also be considered to assess the deltoid ligament
- CT scan very useful for delineating anatomy of more complex fracture patterns

TREATMENT

ANKLE FRACTURES 9-2

Dislocation
- Immediate reduction to reduce skin tenting and prevent neurovascular compromise
- Splint to maintain reduction—repeat X-rays or fluoroscopy to confirm reduction post splintage

Nonoperative
- Stable ankle fractures (no medial clear space widening; isolated malleolar fracture without displacement or tibiotalar subluxation)
- Unstable but nondisplaced fractures that can effectively be held reduced in a splint or cast; patients require very close clinical follow-up
- Poor surgical candidates (uncontrolled diabetes, poor soft-tissue envelope, other potentially adverse healing factors)

Operative
- Displaced or unstable ankle fractures that cannot be held in acceptable alignment
- Goal is restoration of anatomic relationships between the talus and the tibial plafond to allow early mobilization.

- Open injuries should be thoroughly irrigated and dressed with sterile dressings prior to splint application; these are surgical urgencies.

ISOLATED MEDIAL MALLEOLUS

- Medial approach is usually recommended, which runs obliquely along the ankle and is parallel to the saphenous nerve and vein. Incision curves from posterosuperomedial to anteroinferolateral to enable viewing of the anteromedial joint, to facilitate reduction, exposure of the talus, and to visualize the posteromedial fracture exit for reduction and fixation.
- Screw fixation perpendicular to the fracture line (cannulated screws, partially threaded screws vs bicortical screws placed in lag fashion)
- Minimum two screw fixation to allow for rotational stability
- Can be modified with a screw/washer and/or K-wire construct depending on fracture fragment size and/or degree of comminution
- Antiglide plate indicated for vertical sheer fractures
- Tension band construct versus very small screws for distal fractures and small fragments

---

ISOLATED LATERAL MALLEOLUS

- Direct lateral approach over the fibula (disadvantage = prominent hardware) or the posterolateral approach (disadvantage = peroneal irritation/tearing) can be used.
- Direct lateral plate with appropriate bend or anatomic plate
- Consider lag screw placement prior to plate, generally from anterior proximal to posterior distal
- Posterolateral plate (antiglide plate; bicortical screw fixation distally)
- Percutaneous—intramedullary fixation with either single screw or K-wire; less commonly indicated, better for transverse fracture or poor soft-tissue envelope

---

BIMALLEOLAR ANKLE FRACTURE

- Open reduction and internal fixation using the methods discussed above for exposure on both sides of the ankle

---

TRIMALLEOLAR ANKLE FRACTURE

- Open reduction and internal fixation using methods discussed above for medial malleolar and lateral malleolar fixation. As for posterior malleolar fracture fragment:

- If posterior malleolar fragment involves a significant enough degree of the articular surface and/or is sizable enough such that the talus subluxates posteriorly, then it needs to also be surgically fixed.
- If able to close reduce the posterior malleolus, or facilitate indirect reduction via reduction and fixation of the medial and lateral malleoli, this fragment may be amenable to percutaneous fixation with anterior to posterior screw fixation.
- If unable to reduce, or fracture fragment is sufficiently large and/or comminuted, may decide a posterior or transfibular (through the fibula fracture) exposure to aid reduction and fixation.
- Posterior plating to buttress fragment versus screw fixation
- Fixation of the lateral malleolus as described above

PILON FRACTURE

- Often higher energy axial load injury involving increased comminution of tibial metaphysis; extension into the ankle joint is very common.
- This injury is differentiated from other ankle fracture types by virtue of both its mechanism (usually higher energy injury from axial load or impaction) and its "personality" (greater bony/soft-tissue damage due to worse bone/soft-tissue envelope).
- Complication rates are higher and fixation is often more complex in these patients.
- Take longer to heal and usually slower to weight bear. See more detailed explanation below.

ANKLE SYNDESMOSIS

- The syndesmotic ligaments are important because they hold the mortise of the ankle together to keep the talus stable between the tibia and the fibula. They are injured in approximately 30% to 40% of all ankle fractures, and can present either frankly or occultly in nature. High index of suspicion is often necessary for accurate and timely diagnosis. If suspected in a patient, then following fibular fracture fixation and restoration of length, the syndesmosis should be stressed intraoperatively with Cotton and/or external rotation tests.
- Cotton test—under fluoroscopic examination, a tenaculum or hook is placed around the distal fibula and pulled laterally. If there is ≥ 4 mm of tibiofibular widening in the coronal plain or excessive ≥ 4mm fibular motion in the sagittal plane, then syndesmotic fixation is indicated. Distal tibiofibular overlap on the mortise X-ray should be similar to the uninjured ankle and at least 1 mm; any difference should raise suspicion of syndesmotic instability.

- External rotation stress test—under fluoroscopic examination, the leg is held in a fixed position and an external rotation force is applied to the foot. Assessment of the medial clear space is made. However, anatomic studies suggest that this is more effective for testing deltoid stability than for evaluating syndesmotic stability.
- An unstable syndesmosis can and should be reduced with a large periarticular reduction clamp placed with one tine on the medial malleolus at the level of the physeal scar above the joint line, and the other tine on the distal fibula at the same level. Can also use a lag screw technique through the fibula into the tibia to attain reduction. Confirm reduction using fluoroscopy. If syndesmosis fixation is anticipated prior to the case, it may be beneficial to attain a true lateral radiograph of contralateral ankle for reduction comparison on lateral view (measure distance between posterior fibula and posterior malleolus).
- A small fragment lateral neutralization or buttress plate is often used for distal fibula fixation—when required, one can thereafter place at least two syndesmosis screws (3.5 or 4.5 mm) using several distal holes in the plate
- "Set" screws maintaining syndesmotic reduction should be placed 1.5 cm (up to 4 cm) proximal and parallel to the tibiotalar joint
- Suture button fixation may be used in place of screws or in combination with a screw but should be divergent to enable control on both the sagittal and the coronal planes.

ISOLATED SYNDESMOSIS INJURY (NO FRACTURE, JUST LIGAMENTOUS INJURY)

- Lateral approach to the fibula
- Debride incisura and reduce syndesmosis with periarticular clamp versus use of a lag screw technique
- Fixation with suture button and/or screw as described above
- Screws should be placed through a plate or with the use of washers (washers are effectively "one-hole plates"). It is recommended in these circumstances that one also address the ligamentous soft-tissue injury with soft-tissue repair or imbrication to maximize outcome.

ANKLE INJURY

Postoperative Protocol

Strict elevation for 2 weeks following surgery until sutures can be removed, or until the wounds heal. The total period of non–weight bearing (NWB) remains controversial, but there is general agreement that range of motion and partial weight bearing be initiated as soon as feasible. Lengthen the NWB period for patients with neuropathy or diabetes or less stable fracture patterns (comminution, vertical shear, large posterior malleolus involvement).

Perioperative Complications
- Wound dehiscence
- Infection
- Loss of reduction
- Hardware failure
- Nonunion
- Malunion
- Nerve damage
- Stiffness
- Posttraumatic arthritis
- Venous thromboembolic disease

SUGGESTED READINGS

Anderson MR, Frihagen F, Hellund JC, Madsen JE, Figved W. Randomized trial comparing suture button with single syndesmotic screw for syndesmosis injury. *J Bone Joint Surg Am.* 2018;100(1):2-12.

Gonzalez TA, Macaulay AA, Ehrlichman LK, Drummond R, Mittal V, DiGiovanni CW. Arthroscopically assisted versus standard open reduction and internal fixation techniques for the acute ankle fracture. *Foot Ankle Int.* 2015;37(5):554-562.

Hsu AR, Lareau CR, Anderson RB. Repair of acute superficial deltoid complex avulsion during ankle fractures fixation in national football league players. *Foot Ankle Int.* 2015;36(11):1272-1278.

Jones CR, Nunley JA. Deltoid ligament repair versus syndesmotic fixation in bimalleolar equivalent ankle fractures. *J Orthop Trauma.* 2015;29(5):245-249.

PILON FRACTURES

TONYA L. DIXON • DANIEL GUSS • NASEF MOHAMED NASEF

ANATOMY

- Distal tibia fractures—involves weight-bearing (WB) articular surface of the distal tibia
- Injury usually a high-energy impaction due to axial compression, which occurs when the talus is driven upward into the distal tibia; often from a vehicular crash or a fall from a height
- Can also be from a low-energy trauma such as when an elderly patient with poor bone stock falls

Most Common Classification			
OTA	**1**	**2**	**3**
A	Metaphyseal, simple	Metaphyseal, wedge	Metaphyseal, complex
B	Split, pure	Split depression	Multifragmentary, depression
C	Simple, articular	Articular simple, metaphyseal multifragment	Articular multifragmentary

The "A" in this classification is designated for extra-articular fractures (ie, distal tibia fractures without any intra-articular component); the "B" classification is designated for the distal tibia fracture that has a partial intra-articular component (ie, part of the joint is still intact and in line with the more proximal tibia); the "C" classification is for a comminuted distal tibia fracture that is completely intra-articular, meaning that there is no connection between the bone forming the joint and the rest of the proximal tibia in the leg.

DIAGNOSIS

- Physical examination—deformity, soft-tissue compromise, excessive swelling (compartment syndrome), neurovascular status
- Imaging—AP, mortise, lateral; CT scan for preoperative planning—if staged procedure, better to obtain after external fixator placed

TREATMENT

- Open fractures—urgent extensive debridement (may require several) and appropriate antibiotic coverage

- Staged procedure (high-energy trauma, extensive comminution, severe soft-tissue injury)—application of spanning external fixator across the ankle (from leg to foot) to maintain length and allow stabilization of the bone and soft tissues so that swelling can decrease
- ORIF of fibular fracture may be done at the time external fixator is applied, recommended if same surgeon also doing the definitive fixation so incisional plan does not limit anticipated future surgical exposure during second stage.
- Definitive fixation—typically 10 to 14 days (range 0-21) following injury
- Surgical approach is based on optimized access to restore joint anatomy.
- Direct anterior approach—intermuscular plane between the extensor hallucis longus and extensor digitorum longus (EDL)
- Anteromedial approach—direct longitudinal, approximately 1 cm lateral to the anterior tibial crest and tibialis anterior—entirely subperiosteal, external, and medial to anterior compartment
- Anterolateral approach—intermuscular plane between the EDL and peroneus tertius or peroneus tertius and peroneus brevis
- Medial approach—directly medial over the distal tibia
- Posteromedial approach—intermuscular plane between the posterior tibial (PT) tendon and flexor digitorum longus, or medial to PT tendon
- Posterolateral approach—intermuscular plane between the flexor hallucis longus (FHL) and peroneus longus
- Choice of exposure(s) predicated on nature/location of soft-tissue and bony injuries, which varies dramatically for these injuries
- Fixation methods—surgeon's preference; may require a variety of hardware configurations depending on the extent and location of the comminution—which can involve tibia, fibula, or both.

POSTOPERATIVE PROTOCOL FOR PILON FRACTURES

Similar to protocol for routine ankle fractures, with the particular distinction that one must proceed more slowly with pilon injuries because of their severity; usually WB and mobilization are slowed, but the important principles of early motion and WB should be followed as soon as fixation constructs/bone quality/soft tissues permit. These injuries typically take 12 to 16 weeks to heal, and this can be two to three times longer for neuropathic, vasculopathic, or other compromised hosts.

COMPLICATIONS OF PILON FRACTURE TREATMENT

- Wound dehiscence
- Infection
- Loss of reduction
- Hardware failure
- Nerve damage
- Varus or valgus malunion
- Nonunion
- Posttraumatic arthritis
- Stiffness
- Amputation (rare)

SUGGESTED READINGS

Mauffrey C, Vasario G, Battiston B, Lewis C, Beazley J, Seligson D. Tibial pilon fractures: a review of incidence, diagnosis, treatment, and complications. *Acta Orthop Belg.* 2011;77:432-440.

Pollak AN, McCarthy ML, Bess RS, Agel J, Swiontkowski MF. Outcomes after treatment of high-energy tibial plafond fractures. *J Bone Joint Surg Am.* 2003;85-A:1893-1900.

TALUS FRACTURES AND FRACTURE-DISLOCATIONS

TONYA L. DIXON • DANIEL GUSS • NASEF MOHAMED NASEF

ANATOMY

- 60% of this bone is articular cartilage.
- There are no muscular origins or tendon insertions.
- Known for a very tenuous blood supply
  - Posterior tibial artery—artery of the tarsal tunnel (main supply) and deltoid branch
  - Anterior tibial artery—dorsalis pedis and tarsal sinus
  - Peroneal artery—lateral tarsal sinus
- Mechanism—high energy; foot dorsiflexed with axial load

CLASSIFICATION

Hawkins Classification for Talar Neck Fractures		
Type	**Description**	**AVN Incidence**
Type I	Nondisplaced fx	0%-13%
Type II	Fx with subluxation or dislocation of subtalar joint	20%-50%
Type III	Fx with subluxation or dislocation of subtalar and tibiotalar joints	50%-100%
Type IV	Fx with dislocation of all articulations (above plus talonavicular joint); effectively an "extruded talus"	100%

There can also be isolated or combined talar head fractures, talar body fractures (when the fracture line exists posterior to the lateral process of the talus), lateral talar process fracture, and posterior process fractures of the talus.

DIAGNOSIS

Physical Examination
- AP, oblique, lateral and Canale view of ankle and foot radiographs. Canale view provides an en face talar neck view. It is obtained by placing the foot in maximal equinus position and foot pronated approximately 15°. X-ray beam is placed at a 75° tilt from the horizontal.
- Broden view can also be used and is designed to specifically view the subtalar joint. It is obtained with the foot in neutral and the leg internally rotated ~35° and X-ray beam is centered over the lateral malleolus. Four X-rays are taken with the tube angled 40°, 30°, 20°, and 10°.

- CT scan almost always indicated for these injuries to evaluate fracture location, pattern, and displacement; also aids preoperative planning.

TREATMENT

Nonoperative
- NWB in a cast for 6 to 8 weeks with progressive WB.
  - Lateral or posterior process fractures that are minimally displaced and/or <1 cm in size
  - Nondisplaced talar head fractures
  - Hawkins Type 1 talar neck fractures
  - **Note:** If the fracture can be viewed on a plain film, arguably it is somewhat displaced so CT scan always indicated.

Operative
All displaced head, neck, and body fractures, and all large displaced process fractures or displaced osteochondral intra-articular fractures (ankle or subtalar joint)
- Anteromedial approach—intermuscular plane is between tibialis anterior and posterior tibialis.
- Medial malleolar osteotomy may be necessary for access to a displaced talar body or a complex talar neck fracture. Preserves deltoid ligament, which contains blood supply. Anterolateral approach—medial to tip of fibula and extended down to the 4th ray. This approach is used for large lateral process fractures.
- Combined approach (anteromedial and anterolateral) is used to provide maximal visualization to prevent malreduction, especially for complex fracture types such as displaced head, neck, and body fractures.
- Posterior approach may be either posteromedial or posterolateral depending on the fracture fragment of the talar body. Either approach requires careful protection of the neurovascular bundle.
- Fixation—lag screws versus headless compression screws are placed perpendicular to the fracture line. Avoid overcompression as it may cause varus collapse. Bilateral buttress plating is strongly recommended whenever any degree of comminution is identified, which helps prevent varus collapse, restores and maintains alignment/length/ rotation, and permits early ROM.
- Hawkins sign—subchondral osteopenia evident on AP radiograph approximately 6 to 8 weeks; represents a good prognosis for revascularization; valuable for the talar neck and some body fractures.

COMPLICATIONS

- Wound dehiscence
- Infection
- Loss of reduction
- Nonunion
- Varus malunion
- Hardware failure
- Avascular necrosis
- Nerve damage

SUGGESTED READINGS

DiGiovanni, CW, Benirschke S, Hansen ST. Foot injuries. In: Jupiter J, Levine A, Trafton P, eds. *Skeletal Trauma*. 3rd ed. Philadelphia, PA: Lippincott Williams Wilkins; 2003.

Hak DJ, Lin S. Management of talar neck fractures. *Orthopedics*. 2011;32(9):715-721.

Vallier HA, Nork SE, Barei DP. Talar neck fractures: results and outcomes. *J Bone Joint Surg Am*. 2004;86(8):1616-1624.

CALCANEUS FRACTURES

TONYA L. DIXON • DANIEL GUSS • NASEF MOHAMED NASEF

ANATOMY

- Largest bone in the foot; transmits WB force of the leg into the foot
- Four articular facets—posterior, anterior, middle, and cuboid
- Injury caused by axial loading of the talus into the calcaneus (fall from height or MVC)

Most Commonly Used Classifications: Sanders (CT Classification)	
Type I	Nondisplaced posterior facet fx
Type II	Displaced posterior facet fx with singular fx line
Type III	Displaced posterior facet fx with two fx lines
Type IV	Comminuted posterior facet fx

Essex-Lopresti

- Tongue type—posterior facet, despite fracture, remains connected to the tuberosity
- Joint depression type—posterior facet of the subtalar joint is not only fractured but also separated (without direct connection) from the tuberosity.
- Primary fracture line—universal for body fractures; an oblique fracture line that travels through the posterior facet joint
- Secondary fracture line—when present, forms a tongue type fracture when the fracture line forms beneath the facet and exits posteriorly through the tuberosity
- Forms a joint depression fracture when the fracture line exits posterior to the facet

DIAGNOSIS

Physical Examination

- AP, oblique, lateral foot radiographs Harris axial and Broden view
- Harris axial view is obtained with the foot in dorsiflexion and beam is angled 45° cephalad.
- Broden view (previously outlined in talus fracture chapter.)
- Böhler angle (normal 20°-40°)—decrease in angle = collapse of posterior facet
- Angle of Gissane (normal 130°-145°)—increase in angle = collapse of posterior facet
- CT scan is obtained for preoperative planning.

Tongue Type
- If posterior skin of the heel is tented, surgical emergency to prevent skin necrosis
- Beware of the pull of the gastrocnemius/soleus on this fragment through the Achilles insertion; sometimes has to be released surgically to obtain and/or maintain reduction

Nonoperative
- Nondisplaced or extra-articular fractures of calcaneus (<2 mm of displacement)
- Smokers—increased wound complications
- Soft-tissue envelope not amenable to surgery
- NWB in a removable cast or CAM boot for 10 to 12 weeks to permit early ROM and therapy

Operative
- Displaced, intra-articular fractures
- Sinus tarsi approach—extends from tip of fibula and extends anteriorly; ideal for posterior facet fractures with a single fracture line or comminution that is not displaced and would benefit from fixation
- Lateral extensile approach—parallel to the Achilles tendon and curves along glabrous border of the foot; full thickness flaps are elevated to protect soft tissues; ideal for posterior facet fractures with comminution or with ones that require greater exposure to enact more anatomic reduction of the fracture fragments
- Percutaneous—tongue type fractures, extra-articular fractures

COMPLICATIONS

- Wound dehiscence
- Infection
- Subtalar posttraumatic arthritis
- Compartment syndrome
- Nonunion
- Malunion
- Hardware failure
- Avascular necrosis
- Nerve damage

SUGGESTED READINGS

Buckley R, Tough S, McCormack R, et al. Operative compared with nonoperative treatment of displaced intra-articular calcaneal fractures. *J Bone Joint Surg Am.* 2002;84(10):1733-1744.

Gonzalez TA, Lucas RC, Miller TJ. Posterior facet settling and changes in Bohler's angle in operatively and non-operatively treated calcaneus fractures. *Foot Ankle Int.* 2015;36(11):1297-1309.

Longino D, Buckley RE. Bone graft in the operative treatment if displaced intraarticular calcaneal fractures: is it helpful? *J Orthop Trauma.* 2001;15(4):280-286.

Schepers T. The sinus tarsi approach in displaced intra-articular calcaneal fractures: a systematic review. *Int Orthop.* 2011;35:697-703.

LISFRANC AND MIDFOOT INJURIES

TONYA L. DIXON • DANIEL GUSS • NASEF MOHAMED NASEF

LISFRANC

The midfoot can be sprained when ligaments are damaged, but a frank Lisfranc injury exists when there is disruption of the bony anatomy of the midfoot resulting in some degree of identifiable subluxation or frank dislocation of one or more of the tarsometatarsal (TMT) joints. Named after Napoleon's surgeon, who described an amputation through this joint when he witnessed the injury occurring in soldiers when they fell from their horses with their foot caught in the stirrup.

Anatomy
- The so-called "Lisfranc ligament" runs from the plantar medial cuneiform to the plantar base of the second metatarsal, although there are many such ligaments in this region. Their plantar component is far stronger than their dorsal component.
- The Lisfranc joint is composed of the cartilaginous interdigitation between all three cuneiforms, the cuboid, and their respective articulations among the five metatarsals.

Diagnosis
- High index of suspicion is required, because these can be subtle and thus easily missed.
- Physical examination—extensive foot swelling, plantar ecchymosis, pain over Lisfranc joints
- AP, oblique, lateral X-rays (weight bearing if able)—Lisfranc 2nd TMT avulsion fracture (so-called "fleck sign") from the Lisfranc ligament. Need to assess for irregularity or step off of the middle cuneiform with the 2nd metatarsal as well as irregularity between the medial cuneiform and 1st metatarsal, as well as all the other remaining TMT articulations.

Imaging
- On AP foot X-ray, the medial border of the 2nd metatarsal aligns with the medial border of the middle cuneiform. Furthermore, the lateral border of the 1st metatarsal aligns with the lateral border of the medial cuneiform.
- On oblique foot X-ray, the medial border of the 3rd metatarsal aligns with the medial border of the lateral cuneiform and the medial border of the 4th metatarsal aligns with the medial border of the cuboid.

- On lateral, there should be no dorsal subluxation of any metatarsal at the level of the five TMT articulations.
- Comparing weight-bearing views of the contralateral foot is also helpful.
- Stressed radiographs (supination and abduction)
- CT scan
- MRI scan for suspected ligamentous injury (beware as these are non-dynamic tests and can thus miss an occult injury)

Treatment
- Nonoperative treatment can be considered for those who have <2 mm of displacement and maintain this alignment during close follow-up, although some authors argue that any degree of displacement should be indicated for correction/fixation. Nonoperative treatment is also recommended for those with a poor soft-tissue envelope, uncontrolled diabetes, or other medical comorbidity that would prohibit surgical intervention. Nonoperative treatment consists of immobilization in a cast or boot with a period of NWB, followed by WBAT in a boot when it is not painful for the patient.
- Operative treatment is indicated for any fracture or dislocation that is displaced at least 2 mm or shows signs of instability; close follow-up is strongly encouraged for someone being treated initially with nonoperative management. ORIF versus arthrodesis as a primary treatment choice after initial operative reduction remains highly controversial.
- Ligamentous injury—ORIF typically with small frag screws
- Comminuted, chronic or missed injuries—primary arthrodesis with plate or screw fixation

Complications
- Nonunion
- Malunion
- Stiffness
- Posttraumatic arthritis

NAVICULAR

Anatomy
- Articulates with four other bones (cuneiforms, talus, cuboid, and calcaneus)
- A notoriously tenuous, radial, blood supply that worsens with age
- Stress fractures—due to chronic overuse; high risk for AVN
- Trauma due to forced eversion for navicular tuberosity fractures

- Navicular body fractures are caused by axial loading.
- Avulsion fractures are due to extreme plantar flexion.

Diagnosis
- Physical examination; the "n" sign can be suggestive (tenderness to palpation at dorsum of navicular area).
- Imaging—AP, lateral, oblique foot radiographs, CT scan and/or MRI are often obtained in the setting of a stress fracture that is not visible on plain radiographs. CT scan assists with surgical planning.

Treatment
- Nondisplaced fractures—nonoperative management in a cast for 6 to 8 weeks while NWB; if fails conservative treatment, may consider ORIF
- Displaced fractures—open reduction and internal fixation with small or mini frag screws, fix occasionally with a bridge plate
- Surgical exposure must be carefully planned to avoid further soft-tissue stripping and devascularization of the fracture fragments.
- Beware navicular stress fractures, as they have a high incidence of nonunion, particularly when their pathoetiology has not been identified and addressed.

Complications
- Avascular necrosis
- Posttraumatic arthritis
- Nonunion
- Malunion
- Stiffness

CUBOID

Anatomy
Articulates with the calcaneus and 4th and 5th metatarsals and forms part of the lateral column of the foot. Mechanism of injury is either direct via blow to the foot or crush or indirect mechanism via foot abduction and is crushed between the calcaneus and metatarsals. This is termed "nutcracker" injury. It can also occur with extreme inversion, plantar flexion, whereby a far less consequential avulsion fracture occurs usually from the bifurcate ligament.

Diagnosis
- Diagnosis is with a thorough clinical examination and radiographs.
- CT scan may be useful for surgical planning, especially if lateral TMT joint disruption is present.

Treatment
- Nonoperative is recommended in stable or simple avulsion type fractures, with a cast or removable boot for 4 to 6 weeks.
- Operative treatment is recommended for nutcracker or significantly impacted fracture that result in significant loss of lateral column length or instability due to dislocation or subluxation. When indicated, surgery usually requires bridge plating and bone grafting to fill the defect created during open reduction and length restoration. Sometimes bridge external fixation can also be used.

Complications
- Collapse of lateral column
- Posttraumatic arthritis
- Nonunion

SUGGESTED READINGS

Ly TV, Coetzee JC. Treatment of primarily ligamentous Lisfranc joint injuries: primary arthrodesis compared with open reduction and internal fixation. *J Bone Joint Surg Am.* 2006;88:514-520.

Raikin SM, Elias I, Dheer S. Prediction of midfoot instability in the subtle Lisfranc injury. *J Bone Joint Surg Am.* 2009;91:892-899.

Reinhardt KR, Oh LS, Schottel P. Treatment of Lisfranc fracture-dislocations with primary partial arthrodesis. *Foot Ankle Int.* 2012;33:50-56.

Seybold JD, Coetzee JC. Lisfranc injuries: when to observe, fix, or fuse. *Clin Sports Med.* 2015;34:705-723.

FRACTURES OF THE FOREFOOT

TONYA L. DIXON • DANIEL GUSS • NASEF MOHAMED NASEF

1ST METATARSAL

- Largest of the metatarsals and provides greatest stability to the forefoot, although also prone to greatest degree of instability as a result of being an evolutionary atavistic trait through the 1st TMT joint. Stable fractures on weight-bearing radiographs can be treated nonoperatively with WBAT in a boot.
- Displaced or unstable fractures on weight-bearing radiographs need ORIF to restore alignment and medial column stability to the forefoot.

LESSER METATARSALS, 2ND TO 4TH

- Typically fractured through a direct crush injury
- Strong intermetatarsal ligaments provide structure and stability to the forefoot.
- Typically, can be treated nonoperatively unless there is more than 10° of angulation, >3 to 4 mm of displacement in any plane, or multiple ray involvement

5TH METATARSAL FRACTURE

Anatomy
- Peroneus tertius inserts on proximal dorsal shaft.
- Peroneus brevis inserts on dorsal base of the 5th metatarsal tubercle
- Proximal shaft fractures are divided into three zones:
  - Zone 1—tuberosity fracture; typically an avulsion fracture
  - Zone 2—distal to tuberosity, extending into the basilar 4th to 5th metatarsal joint articulation; watershed location of the 5th metatarsal causing delayed healing
  - Zone 3—fracture exits distal to the 4th/5th intermetatarsal joint; typically, the location of a stress fracture
- Dancer's fracture—spiral, oblique fracture of the distal metatarsal shaft/neck
- Traumatic—occurs due to ankle plantar flexion with the foot undergoing an adduction
- Stress fracture—prodromal of symptoms prior to fracture; commonly seen in cavovarus foot; higher chance of nonunion

Diagnosis
- Physical examination
- AP, oblique, lateral foot radiographs

Treatment
- Zone I—WBAT in a stiff soled shoe. Treat symptoms.
- Zone 2—Nonoperative treatment includes NWB for 6 to 8 weeks in a cast.
  - Operative treatment is now considered more frequently to all appropriate surgical candidates and not just to the high-level athlete as was once commonly prescribed. Symptomatic nonunions are recommended for surgical intervention.
  - Intramedullary screw fixation—placement of K-wire is key for proper screw placement; plantar tension plate is sometimes used, especially in the setting of nonunion.
- Zone 3—NWB for up to 3 months followed by ORIF if fails nonoperative treatment. Bone graft is often needed to augment fracture healing, as well as addressing initial cause of the stress (inherent foot deformity, repetitive overuse, etc).
- Metatarsal shaft fractures—WBAT in a stiff soled shoe or boot

Complications
- Refracture
- Nonunion
- Hardware failure
- Infection

PHALANGES

- 1st and 5th toes are most vulnerable due to their border positions in the foot.
- Mechanism of injury is likely due to direct blow versus axial load injury from striking a piece of furniture.

Diagnosis
- Physical examination
- AP, oblique, and lateral foot radiographs

Treatment
- Nondisplaced fractures can be treated with WBAT in a stiff soled shoe or boot.

- Displaced fractures should be reduced and buddy taped to adjacent toe for support; WBAT in a stiff soled shoe or boot.
- Surgery rarely required, but can be necessary for open or grossly malrotated or unstable fractures, or those associated with significant joint subluxation.

SESAMOIDS

Anatomy
- Protect the FHL tendon by being on either side of it
- Absorb pressure with ambulation
- Function similar to the patella and increase the biomechanical advantage of the FHB

Diagnosis
- Physical examination
- AP, oblique, and lateral radiographs, which may include sesamoid view (medial oblique)
- CT scan, MRI, or bone scan may be useful for diagnosing occult fractures, AVN

Treatment
- WBAT in a short boot for ~4 weeks followed by a stiff soled shoe or carbon fiber insert (Morton extension)
- Partial or complete sesamoid excision indicated for cases that have failed conservative treatment; some authors advocate ORIF or bone grafting

Complications
- Cock-up toe deformity from excision of both sesamoids, which weakens FHB tendon
- Hallux valgus—tibial sesamoid excision
- Hallux varus—fibular sesamoid excision

SUGGESTED READING

Cuttica DJ, Putnam RM. Metatarsal fractures: what should be fixed and how to fix it. *Tech Foot Ankle*. 2014;13:177-183.

DIABETIC ULCERS

DAVID C. HATCH JR • DAVID G. ARMSTRONG • NORMAN A. WORTZMAN

DIABETIC FOOT WOUNDS

- **Incidence:** Up to 1/4 of all patients with con (pts c) DM; infection (infx) causes 25% of all hospital stays of pt c DM; precedes approx 2/3 of all nontraumatic amputations (amps) (*N Eng J Med* 2017, in press)
- **Etiology:** Shear forces over areas of prominence or offending item + loss of protective sensation (LOPS) + DM → unperceived soft-tissue (ST) breakdown + bacteria ± ischemia → infx
- **History:** DM, LOPS, physical deformity, trauma or ill-fitting shoe gear; drainage noted on stockings; malodor; poss systemic s/sx of infx; uncontrollable glucose levels

CLINICAL EVALUATION

- **General evaluation:** ≥2 Systemic inflammatory response syndrome (SIRS) pos → NPO now, prepare pt for poss OR pending thorough work-up and eval (Table 10-1)
  - **Vascular evaluation:** DP, PT pulses, CFT; ↓pulses and CFT → NIV studies, if abnormal → arterial US + vascular surgeon consultation
  - **Bedside arterial Doppler:** NL biphasic or triphasic signals at mod intensity; AbNL → monophasic, weak
  - **ABI:** NL 0.8 to 1.4; >1.4 art calcifications likely; 0.8 to 0.3→ mod to severe dz; >0.3 → critical limb ischemia
  - **TcPO$_2$:** ≥40 mm Hg → lowest associated c ST healing
  - **Skin perfusion pressure (SPP):** ≥30 mm Hg pos predictor of wound healing potential
- **Wound eval:** Size + undermining, tracking; base composition (granular, fibrous, necrotic); depth (superficial, subQ, tendon, bone)
- Fluctuance and/or crepitus → NPO now, urgent imaging to evaluate gas/abscess

TABLE 10-1 Systemic Inflammatory Response Syndrome (SIRS) Criteria			
Temperature	**Heart Rate**	**Respiratory Rate**	**WBC**
T>38°C (100.4°F) or <36°C (96.8°F)	>90 BPM	>20 RPM	>12 k/mm³, <4 k/mm³, or >10% bands

Diffuse ecchymosis or flaccid bullae c̄ fascial separation ± copious drainage → NPO now, see Necrotizing infections (**Fig. 10-1**)

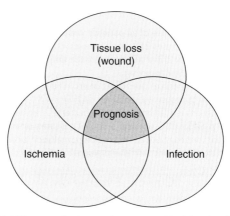

Figure 10-1 Three rings of evaluation and management of the diabetic foot. *Wound Medicine* 2013;03:002

- **Infection eval:** Erythema (nonblanching); edema (nonpitting); drainage (purulent, copious); malodor (±)
  Labs: ↑or↓WBC (<4.5 k/mm^3 >10.3 k/mm^3);
  ↑ESR (>22 mm/hr men, >29 women); ↑CRP (>3.0 mg/L acute reaction); ↑lactic acid (>2.2 mmol/L); ↑PCT indicated in monitoring bacterial infx
  See IDSA Classification (*J Am Podiatr Med Assoc* 2013;103:2)

CLASSIFICATION SYSTEMS

Foot Wound Imaging
- Discuss pt hx, condition, clinical suspicions (abscess, OM, non-healing ulcer, foreign body, etc), other pertinent information c̄ radiologist PRN for clarification and direction in radiograph readings (Table 10-2).
- **Plain film radiographs (PFR)**
  - Radiopaque vessels → calcification of vascular internal elastic lamina and media (Monckeberg arteriosclerosis) indicative of ESRD, DM, also of PAD in the presence of DM
  - Focal bony lysis, cystic changes, periosteal reaction suggestive of OM; ↓ in 30% to 50% of bone mineral conc to be seen on PFR

TABLE 10-2 Wagner			
Grade 0	**Grade 1**	**Grade 2**	**Grade 3**
No ulceration	Full thickness of superficial ST	Tendon or capsule or bone	Abscess or osteitis
University of Texas, San Antonio Note: Wagner + Stage			
Stage A	**Stage B**	**Stage C**	**Stage D**
No Infx	Infx	Ischemic	Infx/Ischemic
Infectious Disease Society of America			
Uninfected	**Mild**	**Moderate**	**Severe**
No clinical SOI	Local SOI >0.5 mm <2 cm erythema	Erythema >2 cm ± deep ST SOI	Moderate + ≥ 2 SIRS criteria

- Diffuse regional lysis osteopenia and intermittent sclerosis → Charcot neuroarthropathy
- Gas in STs → see Gas-Forming ST Infection; poss atmospheric d/t ST deficit, correlate clinically
- **MRI:** Highest sensitivity/specificity in eval ST pathology
  - Focal well-demarcated fluid collections → abscess; if eval for abscesses → order "c contrast"
  - Intraosseous ↑T2 signal → edema
  - Intraosseous/cortical ↑T2 and ↓T1 (edema and bony destruction) → OM
  - Fascial edema and separation → see Surgical Emergencies (Necrotizing fasciitis)
- **CT:** Findings similar to PFR, improved eval of cortices, sequestra; low sensitivity (67%), specificity (50%)
- **Ultrasound:** Rapid, inexpensive eval of fluid collections (abscess, effusions, -"itis") in ST alone
- **Scintigraphy:** $Tc^{99}m$: uptake by osteoblasts, blood and delayed imaging highly sensitive for OM, ↑ poss false-negative "cold lesions"; In^{111} + Ga^{67} useful in identifying OM in pt if MRI unavailable or not poss. (certain pacemakers, adjacent orthopedic hardware, etc), best when combined $cTc^{99}m$, Ga^{67} demonstrates infected and sterile inflammatory ST
- **FDG-PET/CT:** Fluorodeoxyglucose-positron emission tomography/CT scan; ↑diagnostic capability in eval for chronic OM versus differential dz (*Infect Dis Clin North Am* 2006;20(4):789)

- **Wound culture (Cx):** Deep ST cx using sterile technique/ instruments
  - Surface wound swab highly subject to contamination, false results → not recommended
  - Narrow Abx covg c cx sensitivities (sens)
- **Antibiotic regimens:** (IDSA Classification)
  - **Tx duration:** Mild ST infx → Course 1 to 2 weeks PO; moderate and severe ST infx 2 to 3 week total abx (narrowed spectrum)
  - **Initial coverage:** Mild to moderate infx s recent abx therapy → GPC covg, narrow per cx/sens
  - **Initial coverage:** Severe infx, hx of recent abx → initiate broad-spectrum abx including MRSA and Pseudomonas covg; narrow per cx/sens
- **Wound debridement**
  - Sharp debridement rapidly evacuates wound of all nonviable, grossly infected, heavily contaminated, grossly hyperkeratotic, or undermining ST, which is requisite for wound healing (*Clin Infect Dis* 2004;39 Suppl 2:S99).
  - Routine debridement may ↑ healing by 250% compared to infrequent debridement and may ↑ efficacy of wound care therapies.
  - **Hydrolytic debridement:** Moisture (gels, saline, etc) ↑ natural tissue hydrolysis→ mild debridement
  - **Enzymatic debridement:** Topical enzymes degrade target proteins → mod debridement; ideal in pt unable to undergo sharp surgical debridement
  - **Biologic debridement:** Larva therapy, organisms' secretions facilitate breakdown of nonviable tissues → heavy debridement; complex wounds; pts unable to undergo surgical debridement
- **Dressings:** Infx and wound bed prep critical first step (see Table 10-1)
  Iodine and silver topicals used in most all exudative wounds
  Many dressings impregnated c antimicrobial adjuvants (Table 10-3)
- **Negative pressure wound therapy:** Extensive open ST wounds, clean, no OM; any level exudate; ↑ wound perfusion, granulation tissue formation; ↓ bacterial burden, local inflammation, drainage, colony formation, total time to heal
- **Adjunctive wound closure therapies**
  - **Hyperbaric oxygen (HBOT):** pt in chamber c↑ atmos press.; early studies indicated ↑ healing and ↓ amp

TABLE 10-3 Dressing Algorithm			
Wound Type	**Indicated Dressing**	**Dressing Characteristics**	**Dressing Tips**
Dry/eschar/ stable/clean	Iodine; silicone dressing	Antimicrobial; ↓adherence	Poss hypersensitivity to both
Moist	Hydrogels, honey, silicone dressing nonadherent contact layer c moist overlay	Promote moist environment; ↓pain c application and removal	Hydrogels promote anaerobe growth, maceration, pain on removal if dried in gauze; honey poss use in mild ST infx
Moderate exudate	Hydrocolloids; augmented silicone dressings	Mod, absorption.; promote fluid transfer, wound protection	Promote maceration; poss hypersensitivity
Heavy exudate	Alginates, augmented silicone dressings, ABD	High absorption; promote fluid transfer, wound protection	Alginates may be lightly packed into wounds

rates; long-term studies demonstrate similar outcomes with or without HBOT
- **Biologic products:** The use of allograft skin grafts, skin substitutes; amniotic tissue, umbilical tissue, and topical growth factors all associated c improved outcomes compared to standard wound care in many low-quality trials
- **Split thickness skin grafting (STSG):** Indicated in healthy granular tissue s significant depth, exposed tendon or bone, ischemia; ↓ time to wound closure, rates of amp, wound complication rates when compared with standard wound care. Donor site requires wound care postoperatively; consider for final closure of large filled-in granular wound (*J Vasc Surg* 2014;59(6):165712, 46)
- **Offloading**
  - **Total contact cast (TCC):** "Gold standard" offloading; ideal for forefoot ulcerations; beneficial in all plantar chronic foot wounds; nonremovable ↑ wound healing versus removable offloading; applied by trained professional → further wounds poss c inappropriate casting (*Diabetes Metab Rev* 2016;32 Suppl 1:25)

- **Football Strapping:** Wound offloading padding → offload diabetic forefoot ulcerations; healing comparable to TCC c̄ fraction of TCC cost
- Three rolls of 4 in cast pad-1 fan-folded placed longitudinally over plantar foot coursing dorsally, 1 wrapped around forefoot, 1 wrapped forefoot to ankle; Secured c̄ 4 in gauze + coban
- **Nutritional status**
  - **Glucose control:** ADA recommend adult HbA_{1C} <7% (<154 mg/dL); rigid glucose control → reduced risk of limb amp, however, no RCT to date demonstrate rigid control ↑ healing of diabetic foot ulcers
  - **Protein:** Dietary supplement ↑ healing in pts c̄ Albumin ≤ 40 g/L or ABI < 1.0
  - **Smoking:** Nicotine → vasoconstriction to blood vessels including the skin, ↓ ST perfusion; associated c̄PAD, CAD, ↓ wound healing, ↑ wound complications

---

OCCURRENCE PREVENTION AND REMISSION PROMOTION

- **Follow-up care:** See Table 10-2 adapted from Standards of Diabetic Care-2014 (*ADA 2014*)
  Recurrence up to 34%, 61%, and 70% at 1, 3, and 5 years, respectively; annual recurrence up to 58% (Table 10-4)
- **Managing pressure:** Pressure distribution #1 therapy for remission mgmt; >200 kPa plantar pressure → tissue injury and breakdown
  Shoes gear: Recurrence c̄ normal shoe gear >200%; pt c̄ DM and LOPS → diabetic shoes c̄ specialist fit trilaminar inserts. Discuss additional wedges, spacers, trimming, and offloading c̄ prosthetist. Evaluate Q visit
- **Prophylactic surgery**
  - **Hallux:** Evaluate HAV (medial wounds) and/or hallux rigidus (plantar wounds), pronation in gait, consider ST balancing, exostectomy, Keller, joint replacement
  - Lesser digits → Areas of ↑ digital pressure (dorsal or distal hammered digits, bony prominence); digital surgery outcomes in pt c̄ DM similar to pt s̄ DM
  - **Forefoot:** Eval equinus → TAL or gastroc recession; Eval prominent metatarsal (met) heads, consider exostectomy, Weil, or resection; Hoffman → if multiple wounds; Eval pron/supinator tendons → lengthening or tenodesis
- **Mental health considerations**
  - **Stress:** Highest stress during office visit is c̄ dressing change; pt c̄ DM demonstrate ↑ stress levels c̄ normal

TABLE 10-4 ADA Standards of Diabetic Care Classification

Class	Clinical Risk Profile	Frequency	Evaluation Inclusion Details
0	DM, no LOPS, no deformity	Q 1 y	Annual: DP/PT pulses, CFT, 10 g monofilament, 128 Hz vibration threshold, LE reflexes; patient self-care education
1	LOPS, no deformity	Q 6 mo	Annual + Shoe gear eval
2	LOPS + deformity ± PAD	Q 3 mo	6 mo + multidisciplinary referral
3	Prior ulcer or amp(s)	Q 1-3 mo	All of the above

activity compared to s DM. ↑ Stress → ↓ physical activity, ↑sedentary behavior and ↑ BMI

- **Depression:** 1/3 of pt c uncontrolled DM qualify as clinically depressed → ↓ self-care efforts (Lloyd CE, Pouwer F, Hermanns N. *Screening for Depression and Other Psychological Problems in Diabetes: A Practical Guide.* 2012)
- **Cognitive decline:** Pt c DM undergo early cognitive decline, ↓ verbal understanding and ↓ long-term memory scores; accommodate c written dressing instructions and emergency (wet dressings, NPWT malfunction, s/sx of infx, etc) instructions (*Int J Low Ext Wound* 2014;13(4):371)

OSTEOMYELITIS

- OM likely in wound >2 × 2 cm, bone exposed
- **Contiguous spread:** Associated c adjacent wound or infx; m/c polymicrobial, mono poss.; m/c organisms-*S. aureus*; coag neg Staph; anaerobic G-neg bacilli
- **Hematogenous seeding:** Via blood s/p invasive or dental procedure; m/c monomicrobial c transient bacteremia; m/c site → metaphysis of long bones
- **Direct inoculation:** S/p trauma or surgery c bone contact or penetration. Skin flora common
- **Acute OM:** New wound or deep infx, often associated c bony prominence, + probe to bone test → further osseous eval and imaging; ↑ ESR, CRP indicative; WBC/blood cx non-spec

- Hold abx in stable pts if poss until bx c sterile technique. Empiric abx → same as IDSA "severe" infx.
- Bone bx c sterile technique or surgical debridement of infected bone → path/micro eval
- Surgical debridement c residual OM → cx/sens-driven abx therapy, optimal duration unknown, 6 to 8 weeks common.
- Surgical debridement c complete resection + clean margin → abx × 2 weeks for ST infx or c healing s evidence of infx.
- Case discussion and tx coordination c ID specialist highly recommended.
- **Chronic OM:** M/C Hx of wound c prior dx and tx of OM; s/sx may mimic acute OM; often c poorly or nonhealing wound c draining sinus; imaging → extensive lytic changes, periosteal rxn and sclerosis, ±involucrum or cloacae.
  - Follow prior cx/sens; if not available → see "bone biopsy" in acute OM
  - Parenteral abx may be initiated; PO abx in pt c funct gut as alternative; may require chronic suppressive abx therapy in pts c multiple recurrence or poor candidate for surgical intervention.
  - Case discussion and tx coordination c ID specialist highly recommended.

SURGICAL EMERGENCIES

- **Necrotizing infections:** Limb/life-threatening infx that causes acute inflamm rxn → separation of fascial planes, rapid severe tissue destruction; systemic s/sx of shock; high morbidity and high incidence of mortality
- Polymicrobial (≥1 anaerobe + ≥1 facult anaerobe ± Enterobacteriaceae) or monomicrobial (m/c Group A Strep [GAS] and CA-MRSA)
- **GAS pathogenicity:** M protein-antiphagocytic; pyrogenic exotoxins A, B, C→ ↑inflammatory cytokines, proliferation of T cells → shock (strep TSS)
- **Common findings:** ↑↑WBC, often >20,000/µL; m/c >2 SIRS+.; freq uncontrolled diarrhea; may or may not have chronic wound; can start c minor tissue lesion
- **Imaging:** See "Imaging"
- **Intervention:** Rapid identification c early IV abx (IDSA severe) and surgery; add Clindamycin to abx regimen (inhib bact protein synthesis, neutralize exotoxin); debridement c wide resection of all areas of undermining ST and fascial separation (simple digital blunt dissection); Bx for cx/sens/path eval; copious lavage (pulse lavage, often > 3 L);

consider surgical pain pump or PCA; high quality wound care and frequent monitoring of adjacent ST for advancing erythema. Consult ID.

- Discuss the likelihood and consent for amp at most prox level based on clin findings c pt and fam.
- **Gas-forming ST infection:** Limb/life-threatening muscle/ST infx; m/c *Clostridium perfringens*, then *Clostridium septicum*; *Clostridium* form endospores, found in GI tract, soil, marine environments.
- Pt presentation varies drastically esp c DM; significant malodor, ST crepitus and/or fluctuance; + gas on PFR
- **Intervention:** Rapid identification c early parenteral abx (IDSA severe) and surgical intervention; I&D of all purulence with access to all infected st compartments including tendon sheaths. Surgical exploration of adjacent ST warranted. Liberal debridement of nonviable, dysvascular, or infected ST. Copious irrigation, often >3 L of all areas of purulence; pack open; monitor pt SIRS, labs, and wound frequently for advancing/persistent infx (**Fig. 10-2**)

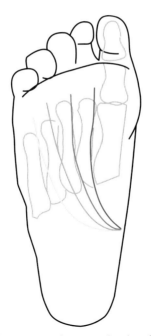

Figure 10-2 Possible incision approaches to access deep plantar foot infections

- Evaluate ST for viability and perfusion in pre-op; discuss the likelihood and consent for amp at most prox level based on clin findings c pt and fam
- **Approach to deep plantar space infection:** Useful in surgical emergencies and nonemergent I&D
  - **Loeffler and Ballard:** Beginning prox, post to med mal, extending distal-laterally toward midline terminating b/t 1st and 2nd met heads (see **Fig. 10-2**).
  - Modifiable → access to multiple plantar spaces PRN (see **Fig. 10-2**)
  - Order: 1. Investigation (size, ST involvement, foreign bodies, abscess) → 2. Debride all nonviable, dysvascular, or infx ST incl tendons, muscle; debride nonviable or infx bone (often serial debridement required) c bx → 3. Lavage → 4. Closure c high quality wound care (see Therapeutic Modalities)

CHARCOT NEUROARTHROPATHY

DAVID C. HATCH JR • DAVID G. ARMSTRONG • NORMAN A. WORTZMAN

- **Incidence:** As ↑ 0.12%, M > F, fifth to sixth decade of life; unilateral Lisfranc (tarsometatarsal) and Chopart (midtarsal) joint m/c, ankle, forefoot, STJ incidences reported.
- **Etiology:** Largely unknown, likely d/t LOPS + loss of vasomotor control d/t autonomic neuropathy + repetitive microtrauma → acute inflammation (TNF-α, IL-1) and bony resorption (NF, RANK, RANK-L pathways).
- **History:** Often misdiagnosed as cellulitis and/or OM; maintain high clinical suspicion in pt c hx of DM, LOPS (infrequently s LOPS), new onset unilateral erythema, edema, warmth (>4°F difference b/t limbs) to diffuse area of the foot. Poss hx of trauma though pt c LOPS often unaware; in absence of infx often no systemic complaint; pt c DM and chronic diabetic foot wound may also have underlying ST or bony infx.
- **Clinical evaluation**
  - **General eval:** See Clinical Eval in Diabetic Foot Wound section.
  - **Labs:** Normal WBC, age-appropriate ESR/CRP in isolated Charcot neuroarthropathy. Concern for OM → see OM section.
- **Radiographic evaluation**
  - **PFR:** Early → ↓ joint space, ST edema; Late → diffuse mottled bony resorption, joint collapse → deformity progression; poss consolidation, sclerosis, bony regrowth in midfoot/rearfoot Charcot; recall ↓ in 30% to 50% of bone mineral conc to be seen on PFR
  - **MRI:** Differentiation from OM difficult; MRI with contrast + finding of fluid collection, fat replacement, sinus tract or extensive marrow abnormality indicative of OM
  - **Scintigraphy:** In equivocal PFR or MRI → labeled WBC indicated; PET CT effectiveness in differentiation undetermined
- **Clinical phases** (Eichenholtz classification)
- **Intervention**
  - **Bone bx:** Isolated Charcot → bone/joint fluid cx s growth; Path s organisms or OM; joint fluid s crystals; often OM coexists c Charcot neuroarthropathy
  - **Charcot + OM:** see OM tx; pt to remain NWB if unable to cast
  - **Bone metabolism regulators:** Bisphosphonates: few studies show promotion of resolution of sx or ↑ bone mineral. Calcitonin ↓urinary by-products of bone metab, ↓ evidence of improved sx or outcome

Eichenholtz Classification of Charcot Neuroarthropathy			
Stage	Phase	Physical Findings	PFR Findings
0	Inflammatory	Sudden onset erythema, edema, warmth	Little to no change
I	Development	Persistent erythema, edema, warmth	Joint dislocations, fracture, osseous fragments
2	Coalescence	Decreased erythema, edema, warmth	Fracture healing, ↑sclerosis, trabeculation, fragment resorpt
3	Remodeling	Resolved	↑Trabeculation, mature bone callus, ↓sclerosis

- **Casting:** Early intervention casting through coalescence and remodeling of plantar-grade foot; x several mos; pt to remain strict NWB if unable to cast
- **Offloading surgery:** Deformity s/p remodeling; ideal for strict plantar prominence; may plan plantar prominence c ulcer debridement or ulcerectomy c primary closure; chronic wound → eval for OM
- **Reconstruction:** Poorly recommended, high morbidity; primary goal to maintain/reproduce functional plantigrade foot and ↓ ST breakdown, prevent amp; s/p remodeling; d/t significant morbidity of ankle Charcot neuroarthropathy consider stabilizing intervention early (frame)
- **Arthrodesis:** Medial column → arch reproduction; Midfoot: Lisfranc or Charcot joint → promote stability of midfoot and reduction of prominence; Hindfoot: STJ, triple → stabilize rearfoot in plantigrade position, ring Ilizarov fixator m/c method of fixation; Ankle → stabilize early c ring distraction/NWB, often severe OA → arthrodesis

SUGGESTED READINGS

Lowery NJ, Woods JB, Armstrong DG. Surgical management of Charcot neuroarthropathy of the foot and ankle: a systematic review. *Foot Ankle Int.* 2012;33:113-121.

Rosenbaum AJ, DiPreta JA. Classifications in brief: Eichenholtz classification of Charcot arthropathy. *Clin Orthop Relat Res.* 2015;473:1168-1171.

Trepamn E, Nihal A, Pinzur MS. Charcot neuroarthropathy of the foot and ankle. *Foot Ankle Int.* 2005;26:46-63.

DAVID C. HATCH JR • DAVID G. ARMSTRONG • NORMAN A. WORTZMAN

KEY PRINCIPLES TO AMPUTATION SUCCESS

- Often an important step to return pt c chronic wounds to WB → improve well-being
- General considerations at all levels
  - Incisions and bone resection should be planned carefully and dictated by infx severity + vascular exam results + clinical findings including poss excision of wounds; Level provides functional foot c optimized surface area to ↓ ST breakdown
  - **"Too few toes" sign:** Hallux + 1 lesser digit or 1 lesser digit + 2 additional digital/ray amp(s) → mechanical dysfunction → breakdown; consideration of TMA recommended (*Wound Med* 2014;4:37).
  - Shoeable amp levels with consideration for social and physical satisfaction c poorly mechanized or mangled/unsightly amp levels
  - Meticulous ST handling during surgery is paramount; close flaps s tension; monitor tenting of ST
  - Osteotomy c power instruments ↓ bony hypertrophy and ulcer formation s/p amp. Met osteotomies should be slightly beveled proximal plantar to dorsal distal, proximal medial to distal lateral on 1st met, and proximal lateral to distal medial on 5th met
  - Transfer lesions: up to 43% of pts acquire transfer lesion s/p digit amp: Met head resection:ulceration → 1st: 69%; 2nd: 44%; 3rd: 52%; 4th: 25%; 5th: 19%; 50% of multiple (not pan) met head resection demonstrated transfer lesions
- **Hallux amp:** Greatest incidence of transfer lesions; easily shoeable; ↓propulsion; consider contracture of peroneus longus c recurrent sub 1st met head ulcers, poss longus to brevis tenodesis to ↓ plantar pressure
- 1st met head resection should include the base of the prox phal and both sesamoids to ↓ fibrosis to met stump and ↓plantar pressures
- Second digit amp alone likely to promote HAV deformity or adjacent digit lesion d/t spacer in shoe gear; ray resection recommended → hallux abut 3rd
- **TMA:** Maintain arc parabola; eval equinus, perform TAL PRN
- **Lisfranc and Charcot:** Poss in select pt; historically ↓ durable than more distal amp

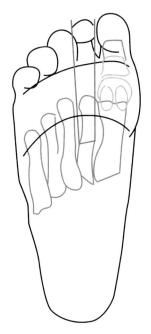

- **Physical therapy:** c̄ resolution of ST deficit, incision healing; include balance, proprioception, strength, stretching
- **Counseling:** Any level amp can be disheartening and ↑ depression in already susceptible population. Evaluate s/sx of depression during follow-up, refer PRN

CORY P. CLEMENT • RONALD M. GUBERMAN

Dislocated hip: Girls > boys, unilateral > bilateral; causes: ligamentous laxity, acetabular dysplasia, malpositioning (breech) (Tables 11-1 and 11-2)

TABLE 11-1 Diagnostic Tests			
Ortolani Sign	**Barlow Sign**	**Anchor Sign**	**Galeazzi (Allis) Sign**
Palpable reduction or "click" or "clunk" felt when abducting the hips while putting pressure on greater trochanter	Femoral head slipping posterolaterally while adducting thigh toward midline	↑ gluteal folds on affected side while prone	Lower knee position on affected side while hips and knees flexed

TABLE 11-2 Terminology of Rotational Problems	
Antetorsion	Internal twisting/anterior twist of head and neck of femur on its own body (39° at birth, 12° in adults)
Anteversion	Inward twisting of the thigh bone at hip
Retrotorsion	↓ from normal angle of internal femoral torsion
Retroversion	Excessive outward rotation of hip, caused by contracture of external hip rotator muscles
Tibial torsion	Inward or external twisting of shin bone (lateral rotation ↑ as age ↑, up to 18°-23° external torsion in adults)
Malleolar position	Angle between knee axis and the two malleoli (subtract 5° from tibial torsion), clinically measures tibial torsion, normal 18°-23° external (*Valmassy: Clinical Biomechanics of the Lower Extremities*. 1996, pp. 136-137)

ETIOLOGIES OF INTOEING

- ↑ femoral anteversion, antetorsion
- Spastic contraction of internal hip rotators (eg, cerebral palsy)
- Internal tibiofibular rotation or torsion (most common cause of intoeing)
- MA
- TEV
- Compensation for excessive pronation (*Herman Tax: Podopediatrics.* 1980:205-208)

Twister cables, lateral shoe wedges (promote outoeing)
↑
Gait plates (when gait propulsive) ← **Treatments for Intoeing** → **Ganley splint** (FF to RF control)
↓
Dennis Browne Bar/Night Splint (6-8 months of age)

CAUSES AND TX OF OUTOEING

- Femoral retroversion
- External tibial torsion
- Posterior position of acetabulum
- Weak internal hip rotators
- **Tx:** Dennis Brown splint, inner heel wedges, gait plates

Genu varum/valgum (*McCrea: Pediatric Orthopedics of the Lower Extremity.* 1985, p. 117)

↙   ↘

Angulation of leg toward the midline, bowlegged

Excessive angulation of leg away from midline, "knock kneed". Presents at age 2-5, corrects by age 5-8 (Normal at birth)

CONGENITAL CALCANEOVALGUS

Most common congenital deformity, prime cause of flexible flatfoot, bilateral > unilateral
- **Etiology:** Abnormal intrauterine position, ↑ internal limb rotation
- **Physical exam:** Dorsal surface of foot in contact with anterior leg, skin folds at lateral malleolus, tight skin anterior ankle
- **Clinical findings:** Foot in extension, slight valgus FF varus, RF valgus, tight Achilles, PF restricted, prominent talar head
- **Pathology:** TC ligaments relaxed or lacking, navicula laterally displaced, external tibial torsion

- **Tx:** Manipulate foot down to $\perp$ to ankle with heel in neutral (5× per correction/3×/day)
  - Casting (3–6 months weekly): Apply BK or AK cast with foot in equinus with plantarflexion of 1st metatarsal and adduction of FF aligning TN joint
  - Ganley splints following casting (6 months)
  - **Surgical treatment:** Reserved when TC angle >30° to 35°

VERTICAL TALUS (CONVEX PES VALGUS)

Rare condition, presents similar to congenital calcaneovalgus at birth but more severe, subtalar ROM key in eval
- **Etiology:** Navicular subluxed dorsally over talus
- **Clinical findings:** Dorsal dislocation of navicular on talar head and neck, calcaneal equinus, rocker bottom foot, supination impossible, FF abduction and DF on RF, anterior muscles and Achilles tight
- **ST path:** Contracted structures (due to DF at midtarsal joint): CFL, peroneals, Achilles, anterior muscles deltoid, TN ligament, posterior ankle and STJ capsule
  - **Stretched:** Spring ligament, TP, FDL, FDB
  - **Osseous path:** Talar head subluxed below navicular, talus locked in vertical position, hypoplastic talar neck, calc in 20° to 25° equinus, abnormal/absent STJ facets, anterior surface of calc deviated laterally
- **Tx: Conservative**: serial leg casting (up to 6 months old), cast foot in plantarflexion, heel inverted with forefoot in adduction with knee flexed 90°
  Surgery: Talectomy, excision of talus head and neck, navicular excision/dorsal wedge excision, peritalar release, TAL, transfer of TA/TP and peroneals, triple arthrodesis, STJ fusion

TARSAL COALITION

Abnormal connection between two bones in back of foot
- **Etiology:** Failure of differentiation and segmentation of tissue mesenchyme → lack of joint formation (*Malay: The P.I. Manual.* 2nd ed. 2008, p. 241)
- **Types:** Synostosis (bony), synchondrosis (cartilaginous), syndesmosis (fibrous); TN coalition (3–5 y/o, less common) CN bar (8–12 y/o), TC coalition (12–16 y/o)
- **Clinical findings:** Peroneal spasm, rigid flatfoot, pain upon WB, stiffness, limitation of STJ motion and possible MTJ ROM, tarsal tunnel syndrome

- **X-ray findings:** Talar beaking, halo effect (sclerosis of sustentaculum tali and calcaneal crucial angle area), lateral talar process flattening and broadening, diminished or absent STJ facets (middle, posterior), anteater sign (CN bar); MRI good for fibrous and cartilaginous coalitions
- **Conservative Tx:** Strapping, foot orthoses, cast immobilization (acutely painful spasm), corticosteroid sinus tarsi injections
- **Surgical options:** Painful CN bars: resect <14 y/o and transplant EDB into void to avoid rigid fibrosis and reoccurrence; pediatric TC coalitions with no secondary arthrosis: resect with possible fusion in future

METATARSUS ADDUCTUS (VARUS)

Common foot deformity noted at birth that causes the front half of the foot to turn inward, foot has "C" shape
- **Etiology:** Uterine position, abnormal insertion of adductor hallucis/FDB
- **Clinical findings:** "C" shape foot (medial concavity/lateral convexity), skewfoot = with heel valgus, associated met primus adductus
- **Conservative Tx:** Manipulation/stretching exercises, Wheaton brace (<1 y/o with flexible deformity), serial casting (with an abductory forefoot force, two sets of casts), orthoses
- **Surgical treatment options:** Flexible med adductus: Heyman, Herndon, and Strong (ST release of all TM joints/ligaments except plantar-lateral, <5 years)
  - Johnson osteochondrotomy (cartilaginous, ages 5-8): Closing abductory base wedge of 1st met and wedge resections of lesser mets with apex medial
  - Children 6 to 8 y/o: Lepird procedure (rotational osteotomies) or Berman and Gartland (oblique closing abductory wedges osteotomies 1-5)

TALIPES EQUINOVARUS (CLUBFOOT)

Acquired or congenital, male > female (2:1)
- **Etiology:** Primary germplasm defect (*George Settle: JBJS* 1963), arrest of fetal development (*Bohm: JBJS* 1929), combo of inheritance and environmental factors
- **Physical:** Medial border concave/lateral convex, talar head prominence laterally, navicular medial, furrowed skin creases along arch and posterior ankle

- **Clinical:** FF inversion and adduction, inverted rearfoot, equinus (TC equinus or tibiotalar), associated with tibial torsion and cavus (FF PF on RF)
- **Types:** Flexible (will respond to casting, 2/2 to intrauterine position) and rigid (resistant to tx, small, inverted, PF calc with posterior leg atrophy)
- **Path:** Medial and plantar deviation of talar head and neck, CC joint points medially and plantarly and below TN, ST contractures (posterior, medial, and plantar), occasional tibial torsion
- **Conservative Tx:** Ponseti technique (most current and common technique): **1st**—Correct cavus (supinate FF, DF 1st met); **2nd**—Correct adduction and varus, abduct supinated foot using counter applied with thumb against talar head, heel not touched; **3rd**—Correct equinus with heel in valgus, perform percutaneous TAL at this stage if needed (*Fixing equinus too soon can result in rocker bottom foot*)
- **Surgical: ST correction** (>3 months failed conservative tx): *Posterior medial subtalar release (TURCO)*—release Knot of Henry, Z lengthening TAL, resect CFL, and PTFL, release posterior superficial deltoid ligament, lengthen FDL; *Medial release*—Section PT tendon, resect spring ligament; *Plantar release*—Incise plantar fascia, first layer of intrinsics, incise long plantar ligament, *STJ release*—Evert heel and intersect interosseous TC ligament, possible bifurcate ligament; after releases stabilize TC and TN joints with k-wires; Steindler stripping, tendon transfers—STATT, TA or PT tendon transfers, TAL

  Osseous (>4 y/o or ST failed): Dwyer, triple arthrodesis, talectomy (severely deformed), Evans osteotomy, amputation (last resort) (Tables 11-3 and 11-4)

TABLE 11-3 Congenital Deformities on X-ray			
Calcaneovalgus	**Vertical Talus**	**Met Adductus**	**Clubfoot**
↑TC (kite angle), ↑talar declination, ↓calc inclination angle, plantar flexed talus	Increased TC angle (>45°), equinus calcaneus, dorsal dislocation of navicular on talus, hourglass talus with it lying parallel to tibia	Angle of met adductus on DP view normally 15°-35° at birth should decrease to 25°	Decreased TC angle, ↑Meary angle (bisection of talus above mets)

Adapted from The Goldfarb Foundation. *The Foundation Board Certification Review Study Guide.* 13th ed. Camp Hill, PA: The Goldfarb Foundation; 2016:267-271.

TABLE 11-4 Common Pediatric Osteochondritis				
Osteochondrosis	Bone	Sex (More Common)	Age
Sever	Calcaneus	Male	6-12
Blount	Proximal medial tibia	Male	Infantile (<6 y/o) Adolescent (8-15)
Kohler	Navicular	Male	3-6
Legg-Calve-Perthes	Femoral head	Male (5:1)	3-12
Osgood-Schlatter	Tibial tuberosity	Male	10-15

DIGITAL DEFORMITIES

- **Polydactyly:** Supernumerary digits (postaxial most common), treatment consists of removing the most peripheral digit until skeletal maturity >1 y/o for cosmesis and shoe comfort
  - **Venn Watson classification:** Normal met with distal phalanx duplication, wide met head (most common), short block met, T-shaped met, Y-shaped, partial or complete ray duplication
  - Associated with Down, Laurence-Moon-Biedl syndromes
- **Syndactyly:** Webbing btwn toes (M > F), most common involving 2nd and 3rd digits, no treatment unless for cosmesis (desyndactylize)
  Davis and German classification: Incomplete or complete webbing; simple or complicated (phalanges involved)
- **Macrodactyly:** Gigantism of digit (M > F, unilateral > b/l), tx (for cosmesis and shoe fitting): epiphysiodesis, amp/partial amp, plastic reduction/debulking
- **Brachymetatarsia:** Shortened metatarsal (most common 4th met), F > M (25:1), 4 to 15 y/o, b/l deformity; clinical signs-plantar fissure at met head and floating toe, Treatment-orthotics, accommodative devices; surgery: lengthening (bone graft vs callus distraction via ex fix)
  Associated with Albright, Down, Turner syndromes, pseudohypoparathyroidism

CONGENITAL AND ACQUIRED NEUROLOGIC DISORDERS

CORY P. CLEMENT • RONALD M. GUBERMAN

CONGENITAL AND ACQUIRED NEUROLOGIC DISORDERS

Spina bifida: Portion of neural tube fails to develop or close properly, causing spinal cord defects.
- **Occulta:** Mildest and most common form in which one or more vertebrae are malformed, no symptoms
- **Meningocele:** Spinal fluid and meninges protrude through abnormal vertebral opening; contains no neural elements and may or may not be covered by a layer of skin, few or minimal symptoms or bladder/bowel dysfunction with paralysis
- **Myelomeningocele:** Most severe, spinal cord/neural elements are exposed through the opening in the spine, resulting in partial or complete paralysis of the parts of the body distal to the spinal opening.
- **Closed neural tube defects:** Group of defects in which spinal cord is marked by malformations of fat, bone, or meninges. In the majority of cases, there are few or no symptoms.

DEMYELINATING AND DEGENERATIVE DISEASES

- **Multiple sclerosis:** Remitting and exacerbating course of multiple symptoms, Charcot triad of nystagmus, intention tremor, and scanned speech, pathognomonic lesion is central scotoma of eye
- **Amyotrophic lateral sclerosis:** Progressive weakness, atrophy, spasticity, hyperreflexia, fasciculations, affects UMN and LMN, wide variety in symptoms
- **Friedreich ataxia:** Autosomal-recessive disorder, cerebellar degeneration, wide base of gait, absent DTRs, ↓ vibratory sense, pes cavus, nystagmus
- **Pes cavus:** Major foot type associated with neurologic disorder, found in CMT, MD, Friedrich ataxia, CP, poliomyelitis, characteristic high arch foot in sagittal plane (**Fig. 11-1**)

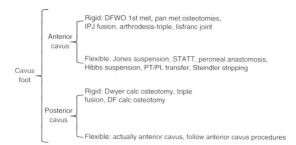

Figure 11-1 Surgical treatments for pes cavus.

MYOPATHIES

- **Duchenne:** X-linked recessive, slowly progressive disorder with proximal weakness in LE later to UE; **Traits:** early toe-walking, waddling gait, shoulder sway, ↓ cadences. **Diagnosis:** ↑CPK, muscle biopsy definitive, + Gower sign-child climbs on own legs to get up from seated position
- **Becker muscular dystrophy:** More benign form of MD similar to Duchenne, progressive proximal limb weakness
- **Limb-Girdle MD:** Autosomal-recessive disorder characterized by proximal limb weakness, more than 20 different subtypes
- **Myotonic MD:** Autosomal-dominant disorder involving myotonia and weakness. Myotonia = delayed muscle relaxation after contraction, abnormal EMG discharges
- **Acquired myopathies: Endocrine**—hypothyroidism, hyperthyroidism; **drugs**—steroids, alcohol, abx; **collagen vascular disorders**—polymyositis, scleroderma, RA, SLE

CNS DISORDERS

- **Cerebral palsy:** A nonprogressive brain lesion 2/2 to insult (usually hypoxia) resulting in pyramidal tract lesion. Types: spastic, athetotic, ataxic, rigid, swing phase ankle plantarflexion (ankle equinus), internal rotation, and adduction of entire limb (spastic type gait)
- **Familial spastic diplegia:** Progressive lower limb spasticity. Types: **Diplegia** (affects symmetrical parts of body; ie, legs or arms), **Paraplegia** (only LE), **Quadriplegia** (all four limbs), **Hemiplegia** (one side of body affected)

- **Brown-Sequard syndrome:** Caused by hemisection of spinal cord, ipsilateral spastic paralysis and postural loss, contralateral loss of pain and temp
- **Charcot-Marie-Tooth disease:** Hereditary motor and sensory neuropathy disorder affecting the peripheral nerves in progressive fashion
- **Etiology:** Most common cause is duplication of short arm of chromosome 17 (gene *PMP22*); molecular signals between Schwann cells and neurons are disrupted in CMT causing axonal degeneration and malfunction.
- **Diagnosis:** Symptomology, NCV, nerve biopsy, DNA testing, "onion-bulb" appearance of nerves under microscopy from demyelination and remyelination
- **Symptoms:** Foot numbness, difficulty in balance, pes cavus, lower leg muscle atrophy ("stork leg" appearance)
- **Gait traits:** Equinus gait with no heel contact, steppage gait with swing phase drop foot, slapping gait
    Treatment: AFOs to control foot drop and ankle instability, PT

SUGGESTED READINGS

Hunt KJ, Ryu JH. Neuromuscular problems in foot and ankle. *Foot Ankle Clin*. 2014;19:1-16.

Piazza S, Ricci G, Ienco EC, et al. Pes cavus and hereditary neuropathies: when a relationship should be suspected. *J Orthopaed Traumatol*. 2010;11:195-201.

INDEX